T0117049

OUR EYES AND OUR VISION

Wolfgang H. Vogel, PhD,
and
Stephen E. Pascucci, MD

iUniverse, Inc.
Bloomington

Our Eyes and Our Vision

iUniverse books may be ordered through booksellers or by contacting:

iUniverse
1663 Liberty Drive
Bloomington, IN 47403
www.iuniverse.com
1-800-Authors (1-800-288-4677)

ISBN: 978-1-4502-9198-9 (pbk)
ISBN: 978-1-4502-9200-9 (cloth)
ISBN: 978-1-4502-9199-6 (ebk)

Printed in the United States of America

iUniverse rev. date: 3/29/11

TABLE OF CONTENTS

ACKNOWLEDGEMENT

The authors wish to thank their families who patiently allowed them to sit on the computer or to study valuable resources for this book for many hours over the past years.

The authors would also like to acknowledge the help received from Dr. R. Clearfield, Bonita Springs, Fl; Dr. Emmons Paine, Boca Raton, FL; Dr. G. Keerl, Duesseldorf, Germany and Drs. August and Gisela Epple, Cherry Hill, NJ. In particular, the authors would like to thank Ursula Vogel, Bonita Springs, FL, and Renate Veeder, Cumberland, RI, who hunted diligently and tirelessly for and corrected misspellings, missing or superfluous words and ill-constructed sentences in this book.

INTRODUCTION

Among our senses, vision is our primary sensory system which we use most. With it, we experience the outside world – we see people, houses, cars, water, mountains, trees, flowers, animals and we also see ourselves in a mirror. Our vision is highly developed and extremely efficient. We can quickly determine the nature of an object we see, its distance and movement and within a split second recognize the gender, age, familiarity and expression of a face (a feat which humans have used for many centuries and which only very recently is now also being used by laser-computer technology, for instance, to identify an individual). We can rapidly judge the speed of an oncoming car or can run to catch a ball thrown towards us. We can also remember the looks of a multitude of people, houses, sceneries, objects, pictures and alike for many years and can even "picture" some of these in our minds even if we do not see them at a particular time. Vision is essential and indispensable to many parts of our daily lives, our work, free time or pleasures. We use our vision to get up and dress in the morning, prepare or eat our food, drive or commute to work, do our jobs, have visual contacts with our colleagues and computers or tools, go shopping, play sports, read books, watch TV and enjoy operas or plays. Vision is essential and indispensable for a normal life – and we take it for granted and give it not a thought until impairment or loss of vision starts to severely restrict our lives.

We use our vision to evaluate other people or objects like "I saw it with my own eyes" as proof and evidence. We often judge the character and personality from the appearance and behavior of a person. Well dressed persons are viewed differently from sloppily dressed individuals. Certain gestures and behaviors might be interpreted as sincere while others as shady but we will say that "we will see right through them" as if they are transparent. A law office, doctor's practice or bank is judged by its appearance and these institutions often try to impress efficacy and honesty with cleanliness and a nice ambience and might institute or enforce a certain dress code of their employees. Facial impressions of other people are seen as smiles, disgust, anger or frustration and will influence our interactions with them. We will treat individuals who smile often quite differently from people who exhibit a sad or sullen face. A smile can dissipate our anger while an angry face can make us even madder and can lead to more arguments or sometimes to a fight.

In contrast, other people also judge us as they see us. Our physical appearance – over which we unfortunately have little or no control – affects our social interactions and how we are viewed by others. Studies have shown that tall and handsome men are more successful in business than short and less handsome men. Psychologists found in simulated or experimental trials that unattractive defendants were more likely to be convicted and received longer prison sentences than did good-looking ones. Pretty young women have a better chance to be noticed and to be married by more influential and wealthy men.

Knowing the value of appearance and the importance of how other people view us, we are keenly aware of how we look. We try to improve our appearance the way we style our hair and how we dress. We select clothes and wear them to enhance our self-confidence and to be better seen and recognized by others. We dress casual when we relax and appropriately when going to work. We choose our cloths carefully when going for an interview to make a good "first impression". Fashion trends are very important to many people and they would not be seen in outdated clothes or shoes - a fact well known to the fashion industry. Women knew the value of beauty for centuries and have constantly tried to enhance their beauty with the help of all kinds of real and magical creams and ointments and colors. Cosmetic surgeons are visited and paid large sums of money to enhance certain bodily features or to change or remove unsightly anatomical parts. All this is done to augment – at least in the eyes of the individual – one's personal appearance which might be necessary to enhance one's self-esteem or to succeed in a job or a business. Beauty, however, is "in the eye of the beholder" and will often change during one's lifetime and certainly will vary among different cultures and over the course of history.

Light and eye sight are not only important how we see others and how we are seen by them, but they also affect our lives and wellbeing physically and mentally. We need sleep and dreams to stay healthy. The light-dark cycle dictates in most cases our daily routines. We go to bed when it gets dark and fall asleep quicker and more easily when the room is dark or our eyes are covered with a blindfold. During the night we dream and dreams are mostly visual images. We dream very little in terms of speaking or hearing or rarely of smelling, tasting or touching. These visual images can be insignificant but can also be nice and pleasant or bad and frightening. After awakening from our sleep, these nightly "visions" can spill over and make us start the day more happy or sad. Looking out the window, a sunny and warm day will stimulate and invigorate while a rainy and cold day will depress and dampen our feelings and emotions. Some people will suffer from seasonal depression during the winter time with long periods of darkness which can partially be counteracted and overcome by being exposed to bright lights for short periods of time during each day. The suicide rate in Alaska peaks during the long winter nights. Colors affect our mood and blue will be pleasing and soothing to most of us while other colors will make some of us feel somewhat uncomfortable and nervous. Studies have shown that prisoners kept in pink rooms were less violent and patients with tremors had fewer tremors while watching a blue light. In 2010, a color chart was developed to study people; healthy individuals did mostly choose yellow while individuals with underlying depression selected gray more frequently.

The perceptions of a particular color, shape and form of the eyes of a person, can even be considered "evil" in some cultures and countries. A person with "evil" eyes can cause great distress and even illness to others and pain and suffering to the person per se. Many customs have been invented by superstitious people to counteract or prevent the effects of the "evil eye" like certain secret hand signals, visits to special persons to lift the spell or wearing of amulets which often bear the image of an eye. An ophthalmologist practicing in a southern European country reported, for instance, that a substantial number of his patients blamed their eye diseases on the "evil eye" of a particular person usually an old woman, a person with eye deformities or with touching eye-brows. This is in contrast to the "good eye" which can not only protect you from the "evil eye" but can also avert bad things and illnesses from other causes. In some rural areas it is still sometimes practiced that a young girl with light blue eyes is brought into the barn of sick animals so that the innocent eyes of this child will cure the animals. Eyes can bring harm and can bring benefit to believing individuals.

The "eye" has even crept into politics and economics. One side of the one dollar bill shows a pyramid with an eye at the top and the words: "Annuit coeptis" and the letters MDCCLXXVI. It was designed by our forefathers so that the eye is to represent the eye of providence which "favors our undertaking" meaning the declaration of independence and origin and future of the United States in 1776.

While we "see" - and are seen - most of us never give it much or any thought how we actually do "see". We take eye sight or our vision for granted – except perhaps if problems arise with our vision. While we accept vision as a basic and essential bodily function, it is actually an extremely complex and fascinating process. In fact, it is one of nature's greatest "miracles". Vision involves not only the delicate structures of the eyes but also to a much greater extent the precise organization and proper functioning of our brains. A multitude of physical, biochemical and electrical reactions occur in our eyes and brains in a well coordinated and integrated fashion to produce this "miracle" of sight. Scientists and physicians knowing this complexity are often surprised that so little goes wrong with our vision – most people have relatively healthy eyes and brains or experience only minor ocular problems. But then major problems can arise once in a while –either from birth or later on in life – which impair or abolish our ability to see. While some of these problems can now be prevented or corrected, some cannot or can only be postponed. Unfortunately, some problems leading to visual impairments or even loss of vision could have been prevented if people would have taken better care of their eyes and would have sought medical help earlier.

In spite of the anatomical, physiological, biochemical, electrical, neuronal and psychological complexity of vision, its basic principles and processes can actually be easily understood even by a lay person. Thus, it is the intention of this book to familiarize the readers interested in vision per se, having vision problems or want to protect their eyes from possible harm and who do not have an extensive scientific or medical background with:

The structures of our eyes and the brain or a wonder of nature's architecture

The basics of our visual processes or how we actually "see"

Ocular problems and their corrections and treatments

How to take care of our eyes

For the reader who is also interested in how our knowledge of the visual processes and ocular medicine slowly developed over time, a brief historical survey is included. It shows how ancient scholars and physicians tried to understand - with the scientific and medical tools available at their times – the workings of our eyes and brains and how to preserve and restore vision through surgery and medications. Their results sometimes advanced and sometimes hindered progress. They were sometimes fighting false beliefs at great personal risks. Science and medicine occasionally progressed straight ahead and at times they got caught in dead ends. This struggle which led to today's knowledge of our visual processes and the high standard of ocular medicine is described in:

History of vision and ocular medicine

For the reader whose interest involves the wider area of biology and who wonders not only how we humans see but how our vision compares with those of animals – sometimes surpassing our own visual capacities - and how it developed during evolution from primitive photosensitive cells to the complex structures of the human eye and brain, a chapter is included on:

The vision of animals

The last chapter will provide the reader who wonders about the future and would like to know what advances are in store for us with:

A look into the future

Again, we would like to stress that no extensive scientific or medical background is needed to understand the essence of this book – only the desire and perseverance to read about the wonders of the eye and the brain and one of their astonishing processes called our "eye sight" or – as it will be shown - better to be called "brain sight". The book is intended to have the reader appreciate the complexity of vision and to obtain information on how to appreciate and preserve this precious gift from nature as long as possible.

The Structure of Our Eyes and Brain or a Wonder of Nature's Architecture

Eye sight or vision is a complicated process which needs the delicate structures of eyes but also muscles and nerves outside the eye to control their movements up and down as well as sideways. Furthermore, vision needs the brain because – as will be shown later – it occurs actually in the brain or "eye sight" is actually "brain sight". Thus, a basic understanding of the architecture of the eye and its associated muscles as well as that of the brain is necessary to comprehend later on the basic principles of our visual processes or how we see the world - and understand visual problems and diseases which can arise and how some of them can be prevented or even cured. Before driving a car it is necessary to understand that the steering wheel turns the car left or right and the accelerator or brakes speed up or slow down the vehicle. Thus, below is a basic but accurate description of most of the important structural features of the eye and brain necessary to understand and appreciate the wonders of our visual processes or our sight.

The eye weighs about 7.5 g and is about 22 – 24 mm in diameter at adulthood. Looking at an eye, only the pupil, the colored iris and the white sclera which is covered by a transparent tissue called the conjunctiva are seen with the two eye lids around the eye. The area above the pupil and the iris is called the cornea which is also a transparent tissue.

The eye **lids** with hairs at the edges consist of skin and muscles on the outside and the conjunctiva – a transparent thin tissue film - on the inside (as well as over the outside of the eye) so that we can blink. Each blink can be controlled by a conscious action but also occurs involuntarily or if we do not think about it. One eye blink lasts about 0.3 seconds and happens about every 5 seconds. Under the lids are various glands to produce tears and this **tear film** (actually the tear film consists of three major layers) keeps our eyes moist and lubricates them so that the eye lids can move smoothly over the eye. The tear film also supplies the cornea with oxygen. Each eye blink clears our eyes of small particles and microorganisms and reduces the risk of an infection. This tear film is constantly produced because it evaporates and drains through a channel on the inside of the eye into the nose. If the tear glands do not produce enough tears, the eye can become "dry" or a "dry eye" results. If the upper lids become too long they can partly cover our eyes and interfere with our vision.

However, a cut through the eye or a cross section reveals a number of other important anatomical structures within the eye as can be seen in the picture below (do not be overwhelmed by all of these structures and names because they will be described and explained in detail later on):

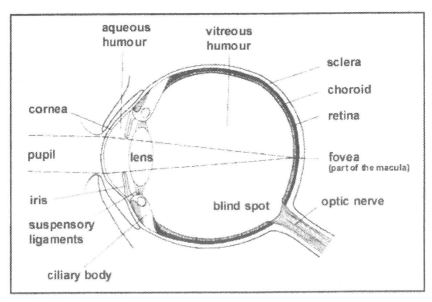

Figure 1

The eye or **globe** located in the eye socket or orbit contains three layers: the outer layer is called sclera and provides structural support to the eye; the second layer is the choroid which is rich in blood vessels and nourishes the eye with nutrients and oxygen; and the third layer called the retina is located more in the back of the eye and this is the structure where we begin processing received images (to be discussed more fully below).

The front of the eye bulges outward and is – as mentioned above - called the **cornea.** It is a clear, transparent tissue without blood vessels – an exception in the body – because blood vessels would block incoming light and interfere with our vision. It is about a half mm thick in the middle and one mm thick at the ends (and actually consists of five distinct layers). Its main function is to properly focus incoming light to the back of the eye. It provides about 75% of this job or accounts for 75% of what is called our ocular refraction.

The next major structure underneath the cornea is the **iris** which is a round or ring-like, colored muscle with the **pupil** in the center (like a doughnut with a hole – the pupil - in the middle). The word pupil originated from the Latin word pupilla or doll – and probably was derived from the reflection of a person as a doll in the pupil - while the colored iris originated from the Greek word for rainbow. Constriction or relaxation of this muscle closes or widens the pupil. The diameter of the pupil can vary from 2 to 8 mm and these changes can occur in a fraction of a second. Pupils of both eyes will relax and contract in unison (at least in healthy eyes). These changes are important in that the pupil functions like a shutter of a camera and as a protective mechanism. By opening and closing it can provide a better focus. In addition, it closes in bright light to protect the inner parts from excessive light exposure and in dim light it opens to allow more light into the eye. Interestingly, the iris and the pupil also respond to our emotional state in that it has been shown that the pupil in most individuals closes during frightening and opens during pleasurable experiences. In addition, constricted pupils are interpreted as aggressive and fearsome while dilated pupils are viewed as warm and friendly. Dilated female pupils have been found to be attractive to males. In an experiment, young male subjects were asked to select a female partner for an experiment from a group of young female subjects. However, one half of them had their eyes dilated with a medication while the others had not. Interestingly, men did choose more female subjects whose eyes were dilated. In the reverse experiment, one half of the female subjects had their eyes constricted with another drug. Men did choose fewer females from this group. Apparently, dilated female eyes seem to subconsciously be attractive to men. This substantiates the medieval custom in Italy of placing a few drops of an atropine solution (a drug which dilates pupils) into the female eye "to make the ladies more attractive". A lady with such dilated eyes was referred to as a beautiful lady or a "Bella Donna" from which the atropine solution later on received its name, namely a belladonna solution (while the ladies might have looked beautiful they probably only saw their dates or partners quite blurred at close range since atropine interferes with near vision). Today the iris whose color and pattern are unique to a person is also used for identification procedures. A picture of a person's iris is recorded and stored. It is good for a life time since the iris does not change after the first birthday (unless it is injured). And the probability that two irises will look alike is almost impossible (for mathematically inclined individuals this has been estimated to be 10 to the 78th power). It is also perhaps of interest that some people and health professionals – mostly in other countries including some European countries - still believe in and practice iridology. Iridology was developed by a Hungarian physician von Peczely in the 19th century claiming that the colors and patterns of the iris represent the organs of the body and that changes in these colors and patterns would then indicate certain diseases. There are charts available which show the patterns of the iris of both eyes with the names of the organs and tissues which they represent. There is, however, no scientific or medical basis of the "science" of iridology.

Around the iris, the eye looks white. This is the sclera covered by the clear conjunctiva which covers this part of the eye but also extends underneath the eye lids. It is nourished by tiny, invisible blood vessels. The conjunctiva secretes fluids and oils to moisten and lubricate the eye.

The next important structure underneath the iris is another round or ring-like muscle called the **ciliary body** with the flexible **lens** in its center (again shaped like a doughnut but this time the lens is in the middle). The lens is located within a capsule and suspended or connected with fine structures or zonules to the ciliary body. The lens is also a transparent structure and contractions or relaxations of the ciliary body can make the lens thinner or thicker which is important when we want to look at an object which is close or far. Thus, the lens is the second most important structure in focusing light properly to the back of the eye. It accounts for about 25% of this job. Loss of transparency or of elasticity will cause distinct vision problems. If the circular ciliary body constricts the lens gets thicker and the eye focuses on near objects. If the ciliary body relaxes the zonules stretch the lens and the lens becomes thinner and focuses on far objects. As a person ages, the lens loses elasticity causing problems with near vision or develops cloudy areas or cataracts causing problems with vision in general like seeing through a veil or fog. Reading or viewing the computer screen for long periods requires constant constriction of the circular ciliary body muscle for near vision which could sometimes fatigue this muscle and cause some eye strain. In addition, you might not blink as frequently during these activities which can disturb the tear film. Thus, it is advisable to look away from the computer or book once in a while to a far object to allow the ciliary body to relax and to blink more frequently to restore the tear film.

The next structure is the **vitreous humor** or a gelatin-like matter which occupies most of the inner part of the eye.

Lining the back and sides of the eye is the **retina** which now receives the visual images. Here is where the visual processes actually begin. The retina is firmly attached to the back of the eye and basically consists of two layers of two types of quite differently specialized cells. The first layer facing the pupil consists of nerve cells and the second layer attached to the back of the eye consists of photosensitive cells. The diagram on the next page shows an enlarged cross section of the two layers of the retina.

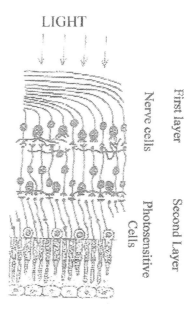

Figure 2

The layer of the **photosensitive** cells (second layer) is divided into long and slender cells called rods (about 120 million) and short and bulky cells called cones (about 6 million). They are very tiny and are only about 0.05 mm long and about 0.003 mm wide. Both of these cells are light-sensitive but cones need a lot of bright light and respond mainly to colors. Rods are extremely sensitive even to a small amount of light but register only gray images. It has been estimated that cones need 3-9 while rods need only 1-2 photons to be activated – with a photon being the smallest unit of light. This is why we see colors during daylight (bright light with cones being active) but only gray during darkness (dim light with rods being active). In addition, cones give us sharp vision while rods are more sensitive to movement. Both of these cells now convert the arriving light waves into a multitude of chemical reactions involving many different photosensitive chemicals or pigments (like the chemical changes occurring in the film of an old fashion camera fixing the images). The schematic drawing below shows the structure of a rod (left) and a cone (right):

Photosensitive Pigments

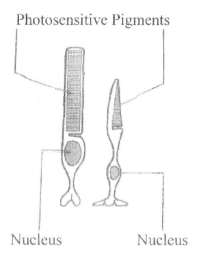

Nucleus   Nucleus

Figure 3

The first or inner layer consists of **nerve cells or neurons** (about 50 million). Nerve cells or neurons are special cells which consist of a cell body and basically two extensions. One is short (as a matter of fact there will be many of them) and called a dendrite and one is long and called an axon (and again there can be more than one). These nerves are excited by certain chemicals which bind to the neuron and produce an electrical current which is conducted along its body (see later).

The dendrites of the retinal neurons (for the anatomical interested reader, they are classified as ganglion, bipolar, amacrine and horizontal cells) are excited by the adjacent photosensitive cells causing the formation of electrical nerve impulses. The axons from all the neurons in the eye are then funneled and bundled into one big nerve called the optic nerve. The optic nerve then extends from the back of the eye (which is the blind spot – see later) into the brain. The optic nerve is essentially a "bundle" of many millions of axons in a normal eye.

Looking at the above picture of the retina one would think the two layers should be reversed – the photosensitive cells should be above the nerve cells or should be exposed to the incoming light first. Why would the light have to travel through the nerve cells first? The reason most likely is that the chemical reactions occurring in the photosensitive cells require a lot of oxygen and nutrients which can only be provided by a large number of blood vessels which are located in the back of the eye. If these blood vessels would be in front they would interfere with the light rays reaching the photosensitive cells. Nature might look strange by placing the photosensitive cells at the back of the eye but nature has a reason and knows what is best for us.

The part of the retina located directly opposite the pupil and along the central axis of vision is called the macula with the fovea at its very center. This tiny area is responsible for our central and sharpest vision.

The place where the **optical nerve** leaves the eye is devoid of rods or cones and is called the "blind spot" and is a small area without vision. This blind spot can be experienced by looking only at A with your left eye closed and slowly moving your head back or forward until the X disappears – X is now in the "blind spot"

A   **X**

We will only see the blind spot if we close one eye. If we would use both eyes, X would not disappear because both eyes do help each other in avoiding the blind spot.

All these structures within the eye are supplied with oxygen and nutrients from **blood vessels** located mostly in the middle layer (choroid) but can also be found throughout the eye – except as pointed out earlier in the cornea and lens.

Before leaving the eye, one process has to be mentioned which is necessary to furnish and control the fluid within our eye and to assure a healthy ocular pressure (intraocular pressure). The **ciliary body** – mentioned above – not only controls by contracting and relaxing the thickness of the lens but also produces the intraocular fluid. This fluid will now slowly flow from this body past the iris and along the cornea (where it supplies nutrients to this tissue) into the corner where the iris meets the conjunctiva. Here exists a system of channels called **trabecular**

meshwork through which the fluid leaves the eye and enters the blood circulation. These channels are very pressure sensitive in that they open when the pressure is high and close when the pressure falls. Due to this mechanism they will keep the pressure in the eye (intraocular pressure or IOP) relatively constant which is necessary for the health of the inner structures.

Outside the eyes, we have different sets of muscles. These **extraocular muscles** move our eyes up and down as well as sideways and allow us to focus on certain objects either near or far or to follow exactly their paths if they move. If we look at a very near object the eyes converge and become slightly cross-eyed. The activities of the muscles of both eyes are coordinated by the brain and they work in unison so that both eyes always focus on a specific object. If they are not coordinated – one muscle might exert more activity than the other – the eyes will become misaligned resulting in double vision.

Up to now, the images of the seen objects have been properly focused by the cornea, pupil and the lens onto the retina which converted them in the photosensitive cells into a set of chemical reactions. These chemical reactions then triggered in the adjacent retinal nerve cells electrical impulses which are conducted by the optic nerve into the brain where the final development of these images will take place (as explained in detail later on).

The brain is the final and most important processing part of our vision. The human brain is located inside the skull where it is enveloped in various membranes. It weighs about 1.3 to 1.4 kg and has a width of about 14 cm, a length of about 17 cm and a height of about 9.5 cm. It consists of about 100 billion nerve cells or neurons and about 50 times this amount of certain supporting cells (such as glia cells- it has been claimed that the brain of Albert Einstein had more glia cells than others which gave more support for his neurons to work more brilliantly). Since all these nerve cells in the brain are more or less interconnected, the number of connections and neuronal networks is way above a trillion. It has been estimated if one would count all these connections and spend one second on each, it would take 100 million years. It is these connections and their networks which gives the brain its extraordinary power. The female brain is somewhat smaller and has fewer neurons but has been claimed to have more interconnections between the neurons.

The brain although often considered to be one organ actually consists of many different distinct parts and areas each of them fulfilling a special function and interacting with each other to complete a certain task. It can be roughly divided into the cerebrum with the "interbrain" and brainstem and cerebellum:

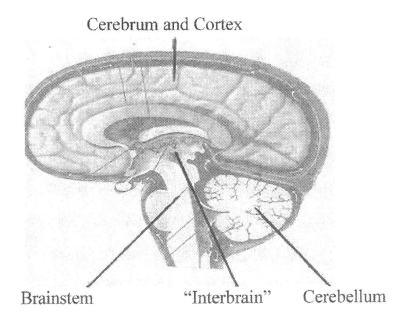

Figure 4

The brainstem contains many of our vital controls and, for instance, makes us breathe and maintains our blood pressure. The cerebellum controls our movements and balance. The largest structure is our cerebrum. It is divided into two halves called the cerebral hemispheres. They are connected by a stalk called the corpus collosum. Although they look like mirror images each of them fulfills its own function. The right brain in most individuals is more concerned with visual-motor skills, mathematical abilities and associations and the left more with speech, language, analytical and logical problem solving. It has been claimed that males generally use more one side of the brain while females more frequently use both hemispheres (which allows them to be more "multitaskers" than men). The cortex is the most outer and largest part of the brain. It looks gray (with a white layer underneath) and derived its name from the Latin word for "bark" or depicting an outside layer of a plant. It is about three mm thick and is folded into many bulges (called gyri) in order to increase its surface area. The mental capacity of this organ is not determined by weight but – among other factors – by surface area to which these folds can add greatly (the brain of Albert Einstein was only of near average weight but there were some differences in the size of certain brain areas and in the folding pattern of his brain). The cortex is the seat of our mental functions such as consciousness, personality, thinking, memory and perceptions of our senses such as vision, taste, smell, hearing and touch.

A look at the brain shows that it possesses mirror symmetry or the left side looks like the right side. And mental functions occur indeed in both sides although both sides are always interacting with each other. In cases of severe epilepsy the stalk between both brains is severed and the individual now basically functions with two half-brains. While there are some deficits at first, most of them can be corrected and the individual will function almost normally. While some functions have areas in both sides others have not. This is evidenced that some people are right and other are left handed showing the dominance of one side over the other. Vision is processed in both hemispheres while some of the interpretive functions are more lateralized. For instance, if a person views a face with his left eye in such a way that only the right hemisphere is involved then this person will recognize the face easier and quicker as when it is viewed the other way around – the recognition area seems to be more prominent on the right side. Speech is lateralized more in the left area and damage to this area will impede normal speech while damage to the same area in the right brain will not. At present it is unknown why this bilateral and unilateral organization of different brain functions exists. It has been suggested that it might provide us with performing multi-tasks (dolphins will sleep with one hemisphere asleep but the other being active which then changes after some time – so they can be always aware of danger and still get some rest).

For vision, the most important parts as discussed in more detail below are: the optic nerve (the nerve basically consisting of the extensions or axons of the many neurons of the retina) entering the brain, the chiasm where parts of the optic nerves from both eyes meet and partially cross over into the other side of the brain, certain areas of the middle of the brain (including the superior colliculus and lateral geniculate body) and finally the cerebral cortex with its primary visual area (area striatum) and its associated visual areas.

Let us start from the beginning. The **optic nerve** containing about 1 million axons all bundled together (like many wires in a cable) leaves each eye through a bony channel behind the eye. As the optic nerves from both eyes enter the brain, it would be expected that the nerve from the right eye would go to the right brain and the one from the left eye to the left brain or perhaps they would cross over completely into the other brain side. The optic nerves, however, do both. As the optic nerves from both eyes meet in the **chiasm,** each of them splits into half. One part of the optic nerve from the right eye goes to the right brain and one part to the left brain. The same holds true for the optic nerve coming from the left eye where one part goes to the left brain and one part goes to the right brain. Thus, we see a part of an object on the left and the other part of the same object on the right side of the brain. While this seems quite complex and unnecessary, this split is nevertheless very important for the brain to process the received nerve impulses properly.

The diagram below shows the pathway through the eyes into the brain with the partial crossing at the chiasm:

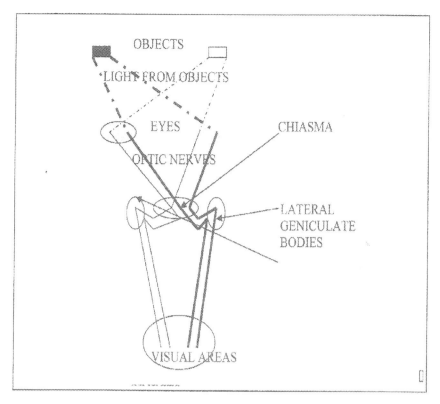

Figure 5

Here it can be seen that the light rays (broken lines) from the objects (black and white squares) fall on both eyes but on opposite sides (rays from the black box fall on the inside of the left and outside of the right eye). From there the optic nerves (solid lines) transport the "images" to the brain. The "images "from the black object (left side) will either cross from one side to the other or stay on the same side so that the "images" are received by the brain on the right. The "images" from the white object (right) will do the same but will now be seen on the left. Thus, only some of the entire "image" crosses while the other stays on the same side.

The optic nerve ends in **special areas in the middle of the brain** or "interbrain" (including the superior colliculus and lateral geniculate body) where the many axons make contact with other neurons which now perform the first tasks of visual processing and also conduct the impulses along their axons to higher parts of the brain. This area is mostly involved in the detection of movements without proper identification of what actually moves. However, it serves a beneficial action in that we can move the head quickly away and protect the eyes if something comes towards them before being aware of what it is. Identification would slow this process and might result in injury to our eyes. We all experience this if we all of a sudden see something coming towards our face and we move the head – while recognizing the object only after our protective movement has occurred. These areas are often called an evolutionary or old area since many lower animals only posses this area and here it is often referred to as optic tectum. It has been said a frog in a container surrounded by dead flies would starve to death because a frog basically can see mostly moving flies.

The areas where vision occurs can be divided into the primary and associated visual areas. They all consist of billions of nerve cells or neurons which are in constant communication with each other. A schematic picture of such a neuronal network is shown below:

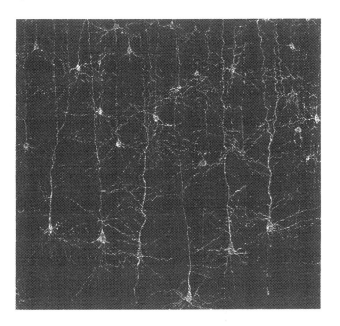

Figure 6

The picture also shows the structure of individual neurons each with a cell body (small white areas), short extensions (dendrites) and long extensions (axons).

The structure of the primary visual area consists basically of six layers of millions of above shown nerve cells which are all interconnected – horizontally and vertically - forming an extensive and complex vertical and horizontal network (Of interest might be that a single gene - called AP2gamma-Gen - seems to be responsible for the proper development of these six layers as has been shown in mice). A schematic part of the interconnections of only three layers of nerve cells is shown below (denoting connections: ←, →, ↑,↓) :

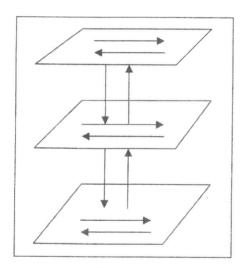

Figure 7

In each layer there are millions of individual neurons which now communicate with each other within this single layer as well as with millions and millions of other neurons in the adjacent layers.

Thus, it becomes apparent that it is not a single neuron or even a lot of neurons but the communication and networks among billions of neurons which finally produce our visual pictures. There are trillions of connections among the neurons and billions of smaller and larger networks. This is how the brain works- using a vast multitude of interconnecting networks.

It is in the visual areas of the brain where we will finally develop the final pictures and will finally see what we are looking at. But just to see it is not enough we need the adjacent associated visual areas in the cortex to help us to interpret and to comprehend fully what we actually see. It is not enough to see a face but it has to be interpreted- is it male or female, is it young or old, is it familiar or not and does it cause a pleasant, indifferent or unpleasant feeling. All these individual processes and how they actually work – and what can go wrong – will be explained later on in following chapters in more detail.

However, the brain does not only receive and see the images of the objects but it is also involved in the initial processes of receiving images by the eye. There are not only nerves which enter the brain (like the optic nerves) but also a multitude of nerves leaving the brain. These nerves control the movements of our eyes and some of their structures which are important to have clear and perfect vision. Certain nerves innervate the muscles around our eyes which control the up and down as well as sideway movements of the eyes so that we can look up or down as well as sideways and can follow accurately moving objects. Again these movements must be well coordinated in that both eyes must move simultaneously and smoothly in the desired direction. Other nerves will control the iris and can constrict the iris (small pupil) or relax it (large pupil) depending on the brightness of the surroundings and whether the object of interest is near or far. Similarly, other nerves control the ciliary body and the shape of the lens in both eyes– stimulation causes constriction of the ciliary muscle and a "thick" lens to allow us to see better at close distances while lack of stimulation causes relaxation and a "thin" lens which now allows us to see better in the far distance. Again, both eyes must respond simultaneously. The brain here functions like a conductor who gives the appropriate signals to each of the players in the orchestra so that each player and section can perform at his best but also that a harmonious sound can be produced by the entire orchestra. All these ocular movements and changes have to occur in unison between both eyes and according to the objects – near or far, bright or dim, still or moving – which we look at.

Up to now, the anatomy of the eye and the brain has been described. But one has to be aware of that all of these structures started out at one time from one single fertilized egg – too small to be seen with a naked eye. This egg contained within the nucleus the DNA or the genetic "blue print" for the new individual. This "blue print" contained all the information how to build a new human body including the delicate and extremely complex structures of the eyes and brain. This is truly a miracle of Mother Nature.

The following provides a quick glance on the development and growth of our eyes and the brain during pregnancy.

Development of the eye and brain occurs quite early on in the development of a human being. After fertilization, the egg goes through a series of divisions producing hundreds of cells which are all alike and which cluster together as a small ball (blastocyst). Thereafter, newly formed cells begin to take on special characteristics and form three layers. One of these layers called ectoderm will give rise to further differentiated cells which eventually will form the brain and eyes (and other structures as well).

The beginning of the eye occurs about at day 20. At age 5 weeks, the eye sockets and eyes start forming. At age 6 weeks two early eyes have developed. At age 3 months, the eyes are more clearly seen. At age 7 months the eyes are fully developed and the baby could actually see.

The first primitive brain cells can be detected after about 3 weeks and will form from there on at an astonishing rate estimated of about 200 000 new brain cells every minute. During the second month, these early cells cluster together and start to form individual brain structures. The lower parts of the brain responsible for breathing and heartbeat begin to take shape. Then the cerebellum and other structures of the midbrain emerge and develop. At the eighth week, the last brain structure, namely the cortex starts to form when the fetus is about 1.2 inches in length and weighs about 8 grams. The head makes up now nearly half of the size of the fetus. Up to this time, all brains – both in male or female fetuses – are basically female or there is no distinction between a female or male brain. However, certain hormones evolve at this time which favor the development of certain brain areas at the expense of others and which form new neuronal connections. This leads to the development of a male brain with its typical male behavior and male characteristics later on. Of course, this leads only to a specific male thinking and behavior and does not affect the physical development of the individual which occurs independent from this process. It has been suggested that failure to complete this switch properly – or that such a switch occurs also in female brains turning them into slightly male brains – leads to homosexuality later on in life. It has also been claimed that at this time some electrical activity can already be detected in the fetal brain. From this time on, the brain grows rapidly and in particular the cortex (which will even develop further after birth, in particular the frontal lobe which will not reach its final size and function until the mid twentieth). The convolutions of the cortex begin at about twenty weeks at which time the brain weighs about 100 g and continues to grow from there on. At the age of thirty weeks, it has been suggested that the fetus starts to recognize and to memorize the mother's voice.

After this time, a healthy child with healthy eyes and a healthy brain will be born if the genes functioned as they were supposed to work and if the in utero environment was healthy and conducive to the workings of these genes. Fortunately, this is mostly the case with most of us. Unfortunately, this is not always the case in some individuals. If genes were inherited from the parents which were faulty or malfunctioning then problems can arise with the health of the child in general and with the visual system in particular. These problems are referred to as inherited or inborn errors and can sometimes be predicted from similar problems in the family tree. Retinitis pigmentosa is an example of a visually inherited pathology. Problems can also arise if the in utero environment is insufficient like during malnutrition or is toxic to the developing child like the use of certain drugs or substances of abuse, in particular large amounts of alcohol. Sometimes ingestion of chemicals from the environment as they might be present in the drinking water and were unbeknownst to the mother can cause problems. In these cases, if such toxic exposure occurs during the embryonic period (roughly first trimester) then the embryo is usually expelled from the uterus. If it occurs later during the fetal period, the fetus stays in utero but does not develop normally and will show specific organ abnormalities.

After birth, each eye continues to grow from about 18 mm (from the front to the back) to about 22 to 24 mm. If the eye ball grows too slow or too fast, then vision problems can occur (as outlined later on). Nevertheless, the major optical and retinal processes of the eye are present at birth and show only minor changes later on until the aging process starts to set in. The eye has only very limited capabilities to repair damage caused either by aging, diseases, disorders or by trauma.

This is quite different from the postnatal development of the brain. The brain increases in weight significantly. Brain weight at birth is about 350 – 400 g while the adult brain weighs about 1300 – 1400 g. This increase occurs mostly during the early years of life and the brain triples almost in size by age three when it weighs about 11 00 g. Adult weight is reached by age 12 years. After age 60, brain weight starts to decline and has lost about 100 g at age 80.

However, it is not so much brain weight which matters but the cross-talk of our neurons or their connections and special networks. Here is where interesting changes occur during our early growth and later on in life. While many of these invisible neuronal networks and their functioning are formed by genetic information – as is the growth of the brain - they are now shaped and modulated by the environment and by learning to respond to and cope with newly experienced environmental challenges and problems. Anatomical investigations revealed an interesting pattern among these neuronal connections and networks. Apparently, after birth neuronal connections increase up to a point where the brain starts to discard and abandon unnecessary connections which would only interfere with newly formed ones. It is like sorting through your telephone book and underlining important numbers and erasing unnecessary numbers which just would interfere with quickly looking up a desired number.

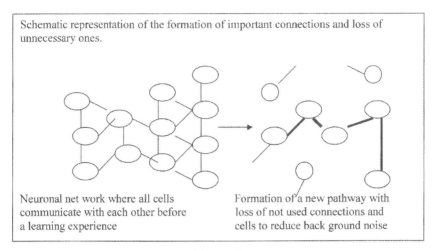

Schematic representation of the formation of important connections and loss of unnecessary ones.

Neuronal net work where all cells communicate with each other before a learning experience

Formation of a new pathway with loss of not used connections and cells to reduce back ground noise

Figure 8

In contrast to the eye, the brain is endowed with a remarkable flexibility in particular at younger ages. Here, it not only adapts to the requirements of our environment as outlined above but can even correct problems caused by faulty genetic informations or inborn disorders. A child born with hydrocephalus (a condition where intracranial fluid secretion is excessive and will increase skull size but decrease the mass of the brain) will show a smaller brain or brain atrophy. This loss of brain tissue results in severe physical and mental problems and a markedly decreased life span. The advent of the surgical implantation of a shunt where excessive fluid is drained from the brain shortly after birth has not only resulted in the survival of these unfortunate individuals but also in the improvement of many of their physical and mental functions. Examination of their brains after death did show that substantial amounts of their cortex are missing but other   areas seem to function quite normally. In one case, such an individual who could see well was examined by brain scans and found to have no visual cortex. However, light which would produce a response in the visual cortex of a healthy individual did now produce a response in a different brain area. Apparently, other parts of the brain were capable to assume the function of the missing visual cortex and allowed that individual to see almost normally.

As an individual starts to age, this plasticity seems to slowly decrease. This was demonstrated, for instance, in 1920 when the cataracts from a blind eight year old boy were extracted. After the bandages were removed he was asked what he saw and he said he saw brightness but could not see a hand moving in front of his face. His eyes were functioning properly but his brain had not formed the appropriate connections with the millions of nerve fibers of the optic nerve. When he was asked to touch the hand, he cried: it is a hand. It took him some time to experience and to learn – or to train his brain – before he could see normally. This shows that the brain can develop the proper visual networks and can "learn" how to see (it also shows that touch apparently helps us in the beginning to see properly). However, when his visual training stopped too soon since he was handed over later on to a welfare agency, his vision slowly declined although his eyes remained healthy. Apparently, the newly formed abilities had not yet been fixed completely to function permanently. At an older age this plasticity seems to decrease further and previously fixed pattern cannot easily be erased and replaced by new ones. In 1958, a blind fifty year old man received corneal implants and for the first time in his life could see. When ask after the bandages were removed what he saw, he said: a blur but since a voice came from this blur he said it must be a person. Again, very long training sessions were required for this man to see more properly and he constantly said that recognizing faces gave him trouble (while it will be pointed out later, that the brain actually has a tremendous potential to recognize faces). Sometimes he would touch an object and would say: now I can see it. Interestingly, he often would prefer to be in darkness and follow the accustomed way of finding his way without sight. Apparently, the old patterns developed during blindness could not be erased easily and the new patterns with sight could not be incorporated efficiently by his brain. And similar cases have also reported that such new visual impressions after long term blindness were often frightening and some of these individuals would say that it would be better to be blind again.

The old belief that all organs in the body can make new cells and can regenerate themselves except the brain is now not valid anymore. The brain can indeed form new nerve cells albeit much, much slower than other tissues in the body. It can use stem cells – these omnipotent cells which can be obtained from embryos, placental blood or other materials – have the ability to develop into any cell in the body. A stem cell placed in the heart will make heart cells while the same cell had it been placed into the brain would have made a nerve cell. It can use its genetic material to form new connections among nerve cells as well as new neurons per se. Recently it was discovered that the brain might use 'jumping genes" – which are genes which are not fixed in the chromosomes as most genes are but can actually jump from one place to another in the DNA helix and can thus offer new ways to make even more unique nerve cells with more capacities and possibilities. Again, the body's own genetic machinery stimulated by environmental clues and stimuli endow that the brain is not a static but an ever adapting organ in our body.

All these anatomical structures of the eye and the brain are important for the next chapters to understand how our healthy vision works, how disorders or diseases can affect our eye sight and how some of them can now be prevented or treated.

Genetic and environment. For the proper development and completion of our eyes and brain we need our genes or our "blueprint" as well as our environment in which we grow up which can be either physical (proper food) as well as mental (education and experience). We have little control over our genes since we inherited them from our parents. Part of our environment is also beyond our control because we could have been born into a wealthy or poor family or in Europe, the USA, Asia or Africa which would have provided quite different social and cultural environments. But we can later on in life choose and change our environment. We can eat properly and help the brain to grow and adjust or indulge in excessive drinking which can damage the brain physically. We can read and educate ourselves and improve our mental and intellectual faculties or neglect them partially or completely. Both of these factors are important in how we see and evaluate what we see. The structure of the eyes is most likely predestined in our genes and the environment plays only a minor role. In contrast, the development and final structure of the brain is basically outlined in our genes but can be significantly influenced, modulated and improved by our environments after birth. This has been shown experimentally in rats. These animals were raised either in an impoverished (only a large, but plain cage) or enriched (the same cage but supplied with various activity provoking objects) environment. When sacrificed, the brains of the rats from the enriched environment contained significantly more neurons and neuronal connections.

Evolution of the brain. A look at human evolution shows some puzzling developments for the brain. From our earlier ancestors, the human brain slowly increased in size over the next millions of years allowing our ancestors to cope better with their environments and to increase their chances of survival. This strategy must have worked well because our race not only survived but increased in size and started to slowly control the earth. But a curious thing happened maybe over the last 20 000 to 30 000 years. The brain actually began to shrink in size from about 1500 cubic cm to about 1350 cubic cm in man and a similar decrease in the somewhat smaller female brain. The question is now: are we getting more stupid? The answer most likely is: no – but nobody is sure why this decrease has occurred. Interestingly, as wild animals become domesticated their brain sizes also shrink. Perhaps the wiring inside the brain has gotten more efficient not needing a big brain anymore. But there is also some good news on the horizon – over the last millennium our brain slowly started to again increase in size.

Summary. For the following chapters it is not necessary to remember all the details of this chapter since the reader can always go back to this chapter to refresh his or her memory. But for the eye it is vital to remember the cornea, pupil, lens and retina which consists of photosensitive cells and nerve cells or neurons as well as the muscles around the eye which control their movements. The long axons or extensions of these retinal neurons of each eye then find their way into the brain as the optic nerve where the two optic nerves partially cross to the other side (chiasm) and finally connect to billions of other neurons in lower areas of the brain and then finally proceed to again connect to billions of neurons in the visual area of the cortex. This primary visual area constantly interacts and communicates with other brain areas called secondary or associated visual areas. It is not just the number of nerve cells which make the brain so special and effective but the existence of an incredibly large number of neuronal connections and networks.

The Basics of Our Visual Processes
or How We Actually "See"

The universe and our world are dark and black. This is hard to understand that there is no light in our world or what we would call light. But there are strange electromagnetic waves around us which travel with incredible speed through the universe (like 300 000 km/second). These waves are invisible but they are all around us (like we know that we have air around us but we cannot see it). If some of these waves – called "light-waves" - will hit our eyes, they can convert them with the help of the brain into light so that we can see our surroundings. Only organisms with eyes and brains make the dark world bright, glowing and colorful.

Now let me cite a perhaps more familiar example which might illustrate this point of darkness and light-waves a bit more clearly (although the physical aspects of this example and light are quite different, the major points are similar): A person sits alone in a meadow in the country side with the cell phone turned off. It is quiet although this person knows that there are millions of people talking on their telephones to each other and that all their messages must fly all over the world. This person sits in the middle of all of this and hears nothing - the world is very quiet. Now a friend calls but no voice is heard because the cell phone is turned off. After the cell phone is turned on, his or her voice is now being heard. Thus, the cell phone converts all these silent "sound waves" into sounds we can hear. This is similar to light in that electromagnetic waves are all around us which are invisible unless we open our eyes which recognize them and convert these invisible waves with the help of the brain into light and people, animals and objects.

In order to understand our visual processes or how we see, we must consider three facts: what is light, how do our eyes respond to light and how does the brain finally allow us to see the world around us.

Light. To start out with light, we must understand its basic "structure", namely what is light and what are light-waves. Just try to picture in your mind water waves with their ups and downs. From experience we know that there are different kinds of waves – sometimes low and sometimes high – sometimes short ripples and sometimes long stretched waves. Sometimes they are slow and sometimes they are fast moving. These waves can be characterized as to their properties by describing their length, height or amplitude and frequency. Length describes how long a wave is and it is measured from one crest to the next crest or from one trough to the next. Height or amplitude describes how high a wave is and it is measured from the halfway point between a crest and trough to the very top of the crest. Frequency is defined how quickly waves pass by and it is measured how often a wave passes by in a unit of time such as a second. The picture below shows waves with different lengths (top waves have the longest and bottom waves the shortest wavelength) and frequencies (top waves have the lowest or three waves pass by in one second and the bottom waves the highest frequency or fourteen waves pass by in one second):

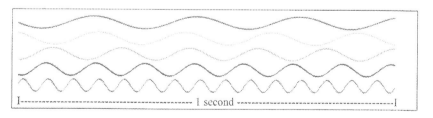

Figure 9

Waves can differ in their length, their height and their frequency (or how fast they travel and pass a given point). Thus, these electromagnetic waves posses all these characteristics except – they are invisible. However, physical instruments (and our eyes) can identify them and detect if they differ in length, amplitude and frequency.

There is something else that fools the eye if we look at water waves. While the water waves seem to be moving they actually are not and water only moves up and down but stays in the same place. A boat in the middle of such waves bobs up and down but does not move. A stone thrown into the water creates waves which move towards you but a floating object on the water will stay in place – just moving up and down. Here nature creates a nice little illusion. As the stone depresses some water and it move down and then up it makes the adjacent water move also down and up and this in turn makes the next adjacent water move down and up and so forth. Thus, the water remains stationary while the individual waves give the impression that they move towards the shore. Another example is the "wave" which people will perform in a stadium with certain sections getting up and down in sequence so that it appears that the "wave" moves around the stadium while all the people will remain stationary in the same place. This is similar with the electromagnetic waves - each individual wave actually remains at the same place but initiates another wave adjacent to it.

To make it easier, in the following we will mostly talk about wavelengths or how long these mysterious electromagnetic waves are. They can occur in all different wavelengths – some are very long (measured in kilometers) and some are very short (measured as a tiny, tiny fraction of a centimeter). And in-between there is a vast multitude of waves of different wavelengths. However, the eye can recognize only a few of these wavelengths. They are quite small or are only a very small fraction of a centimeter long (or they range exactly from 400 - 700 nanometer or nm). These special wavelengths are called the visible wavelengths (which is a bit of a misnomer because even these waves are actually invisible and only the eyes and brain can make them visible) or light-waves. Wavelengths which are longer or shorter can not be seen by us but physical instruments can measure them (and sometimes can translate them into visible objects like the infrared goggles which hunters and soldiers might wear). If all of these light-waves enter the eye we will see white light. However, if only one light-wave (of one wave length) does – like being separated by a prism or by water droplets in the air (rain bow) - then we can see individual colors. These colors will be red (longest visible wavelength), orange, yellow, green, blue, indigo and violet (shortest visible wavelength). To memorize these colors, the fictitious name "Roy G. Biv" (long to short waves) was invented with each letter representing a color – like R for red and O for orange and so forth. If we receive none of these waves, we will see nothing or everything is black. Shown below is a diagram of a prism separating the incoming light-waves.

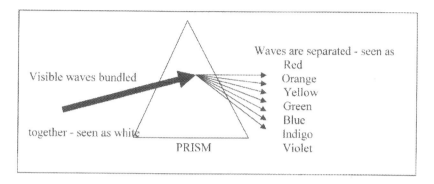

Figure 10

The incoming arrow on the left represents all the light-waves bundled together and is seen by us as white. These different waves will be bent or refracted inside the prism differently and separated into the seven visible waves which we will see as individual colors.

How do we now see objects and how do we see them in different colors? Again, let us stress from the beginning that objects have no color. They only reflect certain waves which we later on interpret as colors. All the visible waves from a light source (sun, lamp) will hit an object and will be reflected into its surroundings including our eyes. If the object reflects now all the visible waves and they will travel to our eyes, we will see the object as white. If the object absorbs all visible waves and does not reflect any of them, then no waves enter the eyes and we see this object as black. If an object absorbs all visible waves except the red waves, then only these will be reflected and the object is seen as red. Figure 11 on the next page is a schematic representation of a white and a red object.

The visual process. The next step is how these waves which are actually invisible are converted into what we call light and what makes us see our surroundings. For this we need our eyes and our brain and their special structures as explained in the previous chapter (the reader can always go back to this chapter to refresh his or her memory).

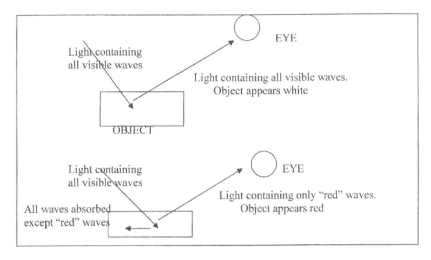

Figure 11

Again, to lay the foundation for what is to come later on let us start with a simple comparative example. The eye and brain function basically like an old fashioned movie camera and projector. The camera contains the shutter and the lenses to focus the objects accurately to its back onto the film where the images are chemically fixed. This occurs in the eye using the cornea, lens and retina. The film is then removed from the camera and sent to be developed to yield the pictures. The film is then placed into a projector and we see the movie or what has been recorded. This occurs in the brain which decodes the information received from the eyes and projects the pictures from the brain finally into the outside world.

The visual process can now be divided into various parts which will be discussed in detail below. First, light-waves enter our eyes where they will be refracted and concentrated on the retina. This is the optical part. The retina converts these waves into chemical reactions and later on into electrical nerve impulses. This is the physiological part. The activated nerve cells transmit this information via nerve impulses into the brain where they will be processed, developed and projected so that we will finally see people, animals or objects. This is the central part.

Eye – the optical part. This part occurs in the front compartment of the eye (cornea, pupil, lens). Viewing the big arrow in the picture below, light-waves – represented by the thin arrows– are reflected by the big arrow. Most of them will be scattered into the environment and will not reach the eyes although some will reach the eyes as shown by the two long thin arrows (there are of course more reflected waves from all points of the big arrow). They enter through the cornea and pupil and proceed through the lens and vitreous to the retina. The curvature of the cornea, the size of the pupil and the shape of the lens now refract or bend the waves in such a way as to accurately project the image of the big arrow onto the retina. This process follows strictly the laws of optical physics and is schematically shown below:

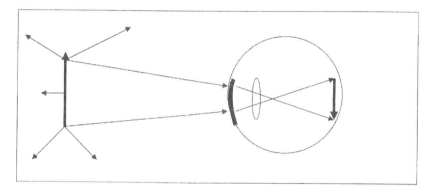

Figure 12

Looking closely at the above presentation one does immediately recognize a problem. The big arrow which we look at is upside down on the retina. And – not shown – left and right sides are also inverted. No problem – we will deal with this later on so that we indeed can see the objects the way they really are and not up side down or left-right side reversed.

The job of the cornea, pupil and lens is to focus the image onto the retina. The thickness of the cornea is fixed and can not be changed. As mentioned in the previous chapter, it accounts for about 75 % of focusing the light-waves or our refraction. The pupil and lens, however, can change. The size of the pupil allows how much light is going to enter the eye and it opens or constrict somewhat if we see far or near.

Its contribution to refraction is quite minimal. The remaining 25% of refraction is done by the lens. The lens becomes thicker if we look at close objects and thinner if we look at far away objects. This is achieved in that the circular ciliary body (with the lens in the middle) relaxes which exerts a pull on the lens through the zonules and it becomes longer and thinner or the ciliary body constricts which relaxes the pull and the lens becomes shorter and thicker. Now the image of the object is accurately projected onto the retina.

Eye – the physiological part. This part acts like the film of an old-fashioned camera where the images are fixed by producing certain chemical reactions in the film. In case of the eye, similar processes now happen in the two layers of cells in the retina which are the photosensitive cells and nerve cells.

First, the light- waves when hitting the retina excite the photosensitive cells. These photosensitive cells are divided into rods and cones. All of the light-waves will excite the rods. However, the cones are more selective. There are basically three different kinds of cones (while all the rods are similar) which will respond mostly to only one particular wave-length. The cones which respond to the long wavelength will give us a red impression, the cones which respond to the short wavelength will give us a blue impression and the cones which respond to an intermediate wavelength will give us a green impression. Again, the individual waves are not red, green or blue but their specific wavelength will only produce a response in certain cones - the red, green or blue cones- and these individual cones will cause us to see later on these three colors. These three colors are also called primary colors.

Well, we see more than these primary three colors – how do we see the other colors? This is done by "mixing" of the responses of these cones. Many of the readers who do some painting will already know that certain new colors can be created by, for instance, mixing two colors together. Similarly, if a particular wavelength can excite more than one type of cone than the two excited cones will "mix" their activities and cause another color impression.

Thus, the three primary colors, alone or in combination, are only needed to basically provide the eye with all the colors in our world.

All the eye has to do is to receive a particular wavelength and either one of the three different cones or more than one cone will respond and we will basically see all the colors in the world. A few examples follow. Long wavelengths will stimulate red responding cones and red is seen. Short wavelengths will stimulate blue responding cones and blue is seen. Intermediate wavelengths will stimulate green responding cones and green is seen. Other wavelengths will stimulate green and red cones and yellow is seen. Other wavelengths will again stimulate two other cones and other colors are seen. If all three cones, namely the green, blue, red responding cones are stimulated, white is seen. No wavelengths will stimulate none of the cones and black is seen.

Thus, a yellow object receiving white light (containing all the visible wavelengths) will absorb all wavelengths except two wavelengths which will be reflected into the eye and will stimulate the "red" and "green" cones. Stimulation of both cones gives us the impression of seeing the color yellow. However, we still do not "see" colors yet. The eyes just register that certain waves have activated certain cones which respond to a particular color and they will transmit later on this information into the brain.

Nature is very efficient – it achieves its goal with the least efforts. We as humans are now imitating nature in that our color TV uses the same principle. The screen consists of an array of very tiny dots of the three colors red, green and blue. These dots can be stimulated electrically alone or in combination and this will produce the beautiful color pictures which we see on the screen.

While this so called three color or trichromatic concept explains most of the colors we recognize it does not do so for all colors. For instance, it can not explain the colors of silver, gold or brown or why we do not see a reddish-green. Here, another mechanism is employed which occurs mostly in the brain and is called Hering's "Opponent Color Theory" (see later). The eyes only work with the trichromatic system which explains most of the colors.

How do rods and cones convert these special waves into something which will help us to see? The first step consists of the initiation of a series of very complex chemical reactions which are slightly different in the rods and cones. For the chemically oriented reader, here are a few hints. These chemical processes in the rods and cones involve a multitude of delicate chemicals among them is a light absorbing analogue of vitamin A or retinal which is attached to a protein called opsin. This complex is called rhodopsin in the rods while the protein or opsin is slightly different in the three cones. Light converts the cis –retinal to the trans- retinal and this conversion changes the shape of the protein. This newly shaped protein causes again certain chemical changes in the rods and cones which now affect the adjacent nerve cells. In the dark, the process is reversed and rhodopsin is regenerated to be used again. A simplified cycle is presented below (although the process is much more complicated and involves many more steps):

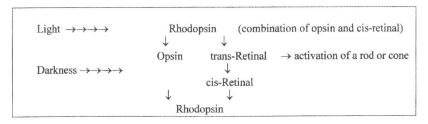

Figure 13

The question can be asked: can we exhaust the capacity of these chemical reactions in the rods and cones. If yes, then vision should stop at one point and we should not be able to see anymore. Under normal circumstances, this will not occur because the chemical reactions do regenerate themselves very quickly. However, under certain circumstances it can indeed occur such as during "snow blindness". Here, too much sun light enters the unprotected eye so that this excessive amount of light can indeed exhaust the capacity of these chemical reactions and vision does stop and blindness ensues. However, closing the eyes for about half an hour allows the eyes to regenerate enough rhodopsin and vision will occur again.

The second step is the activation of a nerve cell by either a rod or a cone. Stimulation means that a nerve impulse is being generated in these nerve cells. Before moving on, the question can be asked: what is actually a nerve impulse? A nerve impulse is a voltage difference between the outside and inside of the nerve cell or a small electrical current which is caused by movements of sodium and potassium in and out of the nerve cell. These changes and the impulses are initiated by chemicals – called neurotransmitters – which are released from certain cells including nerve cells and which stimulate one end of the nerve (the dendrites). This initiates a nerve impulse which then moves along the nerve to the other end (the axon) where again a neurotransmitter is released which then can stimulate another adjacent neuron. These neurotransmitters are necessary because nerves do not touch each other but are separated by a small gap called a synapse. A schematic diagram of the workings of a neuron is shown below:

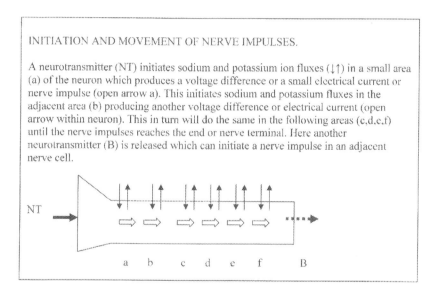

INITIATION AND MOVEMENT OF NERVE IMPULSES.

A neurotransmitter (NT) initiates sodium and potassium ion fluxes (↓↑) in a small area (a) of the neuron which produces a voltage difference or a small electrical current or nerve impulse (open arrow a). This initiates sodium and potassium fluxes in the adjacent area (b) producing another voltage difference or electrical current (open arrow within neuron). This in turn will do the same in the following areas (c,d,e,f) until the nerve impulses reaches the end or nerve terminal. Here another neurotransmitter (B) is released which can initiate a nerve impulse in an adjacent nerve cell.

Figure 14

The following has to be remembered: a neurotransmitter (and there can be many different ones) attaches to a neuron and initiates a nerve impulse (electrical activity) which travels along the nerve cell or neuron and releases another neurotransmitter at its end which can again stimulate an adjacent neuron. These little electrical currents carry specific messages (like the electrical currents in a telephone wire which carry words and sentences).

The photosensitive cells can also initiate nerve impulses in the adjacent nerve cells – albeit they do it a little different as most other cells do it as described above. Here, chemicals do not initiate but prevent formation of a nerve impulse. Rods and cones always release chemicals when not light stimulated which keep the adjacent nerve cells quiet or no impulses are generated (it acts like a brake). If a rod or cone is activated by a light-wave, it stops releasing these chemicals (it releases the brake) and the adjacent neurons start to form nerve impulses. These nerve impulses then travel to the brain where they will be processed further.

It has to be recognized that each photosensitive cell - that is each rod or cone - will only receive a tiny fraction of the outside object and will transmit this fragment to its adjacent neuron which will then sent it to the brain. For instance, a line is received by many rods and each rod transmits only a tiny fragment of the line to its adjacent neurons (the assembly back to the line will occur in the brain – see later). These nerve impulses travel extremely fast along their axons from the eye through the optic nerve into the brain and their speed has been estimated to be between 1 and 100 m per second.

How can nerve impulses or electrical currents transmit pictures? This is not hard to understand because we use it everyday. Just think of your television hooked up to a cable. The pictures you see are electrical currents flowing through your cable into your TV which converts these electrical impulses into pictures on your screen (more recently optic fibers are doing these jobs).

Up to recently, it was assumed that these nerve cells in our eyes only collect visual information which is then transported later on to the brain for interpretation. Recently, it was discovered that these cells already might be able to make important decisions. In mice it was found that certain cells in the retina respond selectively to movement and are activated more rapidly by fast moving objects than other cells. This would shorten the reaction time of the mouse in case a predator approaches and increases its chance to escape by now sending this information to the brain quicker which can now immediately initiate an escape maneuver. At present we do not know if humans possess similar cells but it can be assumed that we do.

Brain - the central part. Up to this point – in spite of the precise refraction in the eye and its projection onto the retina, a multitude of photochemical processes occurring at rapid successions in the rods and cones and the initiation of millions and millions of nerve impulses in the retinal neurons – we still do not see the outside world. Or, in analogy to the camera, the images are still undeveloped in the film which has to be transported to the developer or in this case to the brain in order to be finally developed before we can see them. The developing of the images into real pictures occurs now in the brain due to – as yet largely unknown and in many cases only speculative – nervous activities. What is known is that neurons are always active, constantly creating and conducting electrical impulses and for ever being in communication with each other in immensely large neuronal network. These networks finally produce the actual picture and project it into the world around us. This always means that nerve impulses travel along these neurons which at their ends release neurotransmitters onto other neurons which now initiate their own nerve impulses. Similar to our electrical networks were electricity flows in wires over long distances (neurons) and is channeled by switches (neurotransmitters) into other systems until it reaches our homes where again it is directed into different rooms. All these electrical wires and switches form a tremendous large network all over the country – while in our case everything is packed tightly into certain areas in the brain where billions of neurons exhibit electrical activity and transmit them with the help of neurotransmitters to each other. It has been estimated that we have more than 100 billion neurons in our brain and if each neuron makes connections with about 10 000 other neurons then the number of connections in the brain is about 1 000 000 000 000 000. Thoughts, emotions, sensations including vision are created by the interaction of these networks and circuits in our brain within a split second. This biological network and its results are a true miracle of nature!

The efficiency of these networks can perhaps be visualized by the following example. Six people have to make a joint decision and since they are located at different places have to communicate by telephone. One person, however, can only talk to one person at a time. So each person now calls one other person and discusses the problem and then calls another person to further discuss the problem and so forth. Finally, after many phone calls and most likely repeat phone calls to further clarify matters and many hours spent on the telephone one person finally summarizes the results heard from the other five individuals–

unfortunately, this person might summarize what he or she had heard from the other five people but some of it might be his or her interpretation and might not be quite accurate. Thus, the final summary has taken a long time and most likely contains some misunderstandings, false interpretations and errors. Now image a conference call, where all of the six people can talk to each other at the same time and all hear what one has to say simultaneously. The summary of the discussion is then also heard by everyone and can be approved for accuracy by the group. This not only occurs at a much, much shorter time but also produces an accurate summary of the discussion. This is similar to the workings of the neurons in our brain which are on a constant conference call – except on a much, much larger and faster scale.

While this sounds quite complex, it is most important to remember that it is based on a simple process – a neurotransmitter causes a nerve impulse or small electrical current in a neuron which travels along the neuron and releases another neurotransmitter at its end. This transmits the message to many other neurons.

Now back to vision which also uses this basic principle. As pointed out, the brain receives the information from both of our eyes via nerve impulses. However, it relies more heavily only on one of the two eyes. This is called the dominant eye or ocular dominance. The other eye helps but most of our vision occurs with the dominant eye. This can be easily demonstrated by using your outstretched arm and your hand held in a fist but with your thumb up. Focus the thumb with both eyes open into a corner of the ceiling. Then close one of the eyes and the thumb will stay or move. If it stays the open eye is the dominant one while if it moves this eye is the subordinate one. If the right eye is dominant then the thumb will stay when the left eye is closed and move when the right is closed and the left is open. A piece of paper with a small hole will also show you the dominance. Look through the hole at an object with both eyes open and then –keeping the object in sight – bring the paper close to your face. It will stop at your dominant eye. Thus, most information of our world is received by both eyes and transmitted to the brain which now will rely mostly on the information of the dominant eye and will use the information from the other eye only as a help (like in judging distance as discussed below). About 66%

of the population has right eye dominance with the rest either showing left eye dominance or use both eyes equally well.

Now back to the electrical impulses traveling along the optic nerve from the eyes into the brain. The images received by the retina (where they were converted from light energy into chemical reactions and finally into nerve or electrical impulses) are now transported by individual neurons as bits and pieces to the brain where they will be processed. This is similar to the telephone where spoken words are transformed into electrical impulses which are transported via wires to another telephone which then converts them back into words. These nerve impulses with all their individual informations now travel through many different brain areas where each brain area performs its particular job so that we can actually and finally "see". These areas – as mentioned in the previous chapter - have special names like chiasm (where some of the nerve fibers cross into the other side of the brain), the lateral geniculate nucleus and optic tectum (parts of the midbrain which was developed first in lower animals and is often referred to as an older part of the brain) and the primary visual cortex or V1 area of the brain where most of our sight occurs. In addition, adjacent areas, the associative visual areas, assist in interpreting the formed image and giving it meaning.

In general, these final central steps in our sight can be arbitrarily divided into three major components such as sight location, sight recognition and sight interpretation. They are selectively performed by individual brain areas which work either in sequence or in cooperation with each other. It has been estimated that about 35% of the brain is devoted to vision and its interpretation.

Sight location occurs at the mid brain level. Here is where sight is first processed but only as a sight without meaning. We see something moving before we know that it is moving. It is a common experience that we will jerk our heads back if something approaches our eyes before we actually know what it is. This quick reaction functions mostly as a protective mechanism to safeguard our eyes from being injured. It must occur very fast and a subsequent identification processes would have slowed down our protective movements and the eyes might have gotten hurt. This response is an inborn or innate response. Lower animals like reptiles rely mostly on this process and might eat something without actually identifying what it is.

<u>Sight recognition</u> occurs mostly in the visual cortex (but might involve other brain areas as well) and is the dominant process in higher animals and humans. The visual cortex consists of many small and distinct areas each of which performs a specific task.

First, the information received from the eyes consists of millions of individual nerve impulses (from all the individual light stimulated rods and cones and their adjacent neurons which only contain a small part of the perceived picture) which must now be put together or assembled (like individual pieces of a puzzle). This is done by networking in that each neuron adds its information to the information of other neurons. From these individual dots, networks construct lines and curves and other neurons take these and assemble squares, triangles and circles and other neurons place these into more complex figures until the final picture is assembled. This occurs with incredible speed - as we all know - the moment we lay eyes on an object we see it. Studies in cats have shown that it takes the brain about 10 milliseconds or a hundreds of a second to assemble a complete meaningful picture of an object. Below is a schematic, simplified representation of how we see a house being assembled from individual pieces in different areas of the brain: individual dots from individual neurons in the eye are assembled into lines and squares by individual neuronal networks in the visual cortex and these are communicated to other neuronal networks which finally assemble the house.

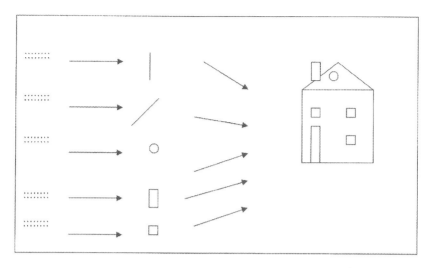

Figure 15

These processes often involve areas of both sides of the brain in order to assemble the true picture. One side might pay attention to details while the other side is only concerned with the over-all picture. Both together construct then the true image. This has been deduced from tests on individuals with healthy and stroke damaged brains. These individuals where shown a picture and asked to redraw it. For example, if they would have been shown a picture of three columns each consisting of 10 As the healthy individual would redraw it accurately. The individual with right brain damage would draw a few As but in a scrambled way. The individual with left brain damage would only draw three vertical lines. This shows how one side uses details (left side sees all the As but not in order) while the other side looks at the over-all picture (right side sees the arrangement of the As in three columns) while both are fused together in the healthy brain to assemble the true image.

A neat little trick to show how the brain fuses two separate lines together is by looking at the two lines shown below and then holding a pencil between the eyes and the lines. When looking at the tip of the pencil (it might have to be moved slightly back and forth) the lines might form a cross:

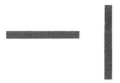

Figure 16

When assembling an object, the brain follows a set of rules. It has a tendency to "image and organize" received individual inputs. A square of As would be seen as a square but also as rows and columns of As. Just draw 5 rows of As and you will see the square and the rows and columns – although it basically is only a bunch of As.

Sometimes the brain after 'thinking" it knows the entire picture will do some short cuts like in the following example:

A

BIRD

IN THE

THE BUSH

Some individuals will read the sentence without paying much attention to the fact that the word THE is written twice since a reader after reading " A BIRD IN THE " and seeing the Word "BUSH" immediately assumes from memory the meaning without noticing the second THE.

Sometimes the brain has trouble to properly identify certain letters or words in a sentence. Read the following sentence and count how many f are in the sentence:

"The beautiful fur of the lady who is the wife of a friend was recently stolen but luckily found soon."

If you count seven fs you are a genius because most brains have trouble with properly seeing the word *of*.

Sometimes the brain will overreact in its assembly and will create images which actually are not present. In the picture below we will see a gray triangle although no such triangle is marked or could be detected by an optical instrument:

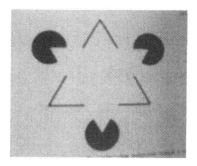

Figure 17

But in general the brain is extremely efficient and gets it right in the vast majority of cases. Thus, the assembly of the image in the brain has been completed.

Second, the images received and assembled by the brain are reversed and inverted (because the light rays in the eyes cross). This is what has to be learned to convert them into the actual seen outward appearance. This is often accomplished with the help of touch. This occurs usually at a very young age (and touch has been suggested is the first sense a newborn starts to use) but sometimes can take a long time in some individuals. A seven year old buy was described who would draw a candle up-site down – and when asked why he would do so, said that is how he saw the candle. Within a short period of time and some instructions the boy would draw the candle correctly. Some of us might also have noticed in our children that a few would write numbers and letters inverted and would have to be told to do it the other way. Of course, the eye receives objects inverted and reversed.

This process is most likely inborn but we have to learn how to use it. Touch and experience will help to interpret what we see correctly. This was nicely demonstrated in an experiment performed in 1896. Subjects were fitted with lenses which showed them the world up side down and which they had to wear consistently. At first the subjects had great trouble walking and identifying objects because everything was upside down. But after a few days of wearing such lenses, they could do so easily and they reported that things looked "normal" again. Then the lenses were removed and the subjects again saw the world up side down until a few days had passed and the world again looked "normal". This shows not only that this is a learned process but that the brain can adopt rather quickly and even at an adult age. Thus, the brain simply reverses and inverts all received images to obtain the true picture (to be in agreement with other sensations like touch which will tell the brain that the head of a standing figurine is on the top). Thus, the conversion problem has been solved.

Third, the brain has to convert all the visual information which arrives in the brain as two dimensional or flat information into three dimensional images because the world is three dimensional. This is helped by using both of our eyes. Objects are seen a tiny bit different with each eye (because the eyes are about 2-3 inches apart) and each of our eyes now sends its own slightly different image to the brain. The brain combines the two images and from the tiny differences between the two makes a three-dimensional stereo picture. This has been used in an instrument called a stereoscope where the same two flat pictures are viewed through the stereoscope at a slightly different angle and a three dimensional picture is seen. Touch also tells the brain that an object is a body even if the brain receives it as a two dimensional image. This was already demonstrated in 1728. An English physician removed the cataracts from the eyes of a 13 year old boy who practically could now see for the first time in his life. This physician reported that the boy saw all bodies flat at first – like paintings - but after some time by touching them he found out that they were actual three dimensional and started to actually see them now this way. Touch teaches proper sight. Thus, three dimensional vision is best in people with two functioning eyes and not as good in people who only have the use of one eye. Nevertheless, such individuals can train their brains to see in a three dimensional way. The examples below demonstrate the brains ability to create three dimensional pictures. When touching the drawing A, the fingers will feel it to be absolutely flat but when looking at it closely a three dimensional cube will be seen. The brain can also be coaxed into the three dimensional mode. Figure B looks like a flat or two dimensional drawing until you want to see a cube – and looking for it you indeed will see a cube:

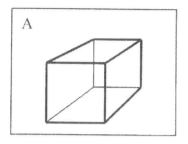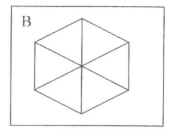

Figure 18

Now you can test your three dimensional vision: center your nose over the black x and look at it. Place one of your thumbs in front of your nose and focus on the black x - you should see two thumbs with the dot in the middle. Focus on the thumb - you should see two dots with the thumb in the middle. Then try it with one eye (while the other is closed) – it will not work and only one dot or thumb are seen.

X

Thus, the conversion of flat into three dimensional pictures has also been solved.

Fourth, the brain now has to add colors to the object if they are indeed colored. The cones do not perceive color but each cone selectively activates its adjacent nerves to create electrical impulses which will travel to the brain and be received by special areas. They provide us with colors. As mentioned before, input from cones which respond to a long wavelength is now interpreted as red while input from cones which respond to a short wavelength is interpreted as blue. Combined input from cones which respond to intermediate (green) and long (red) wave lengths will be interpreted as yellow. This explains the major part of our color vision. However, the trichromatic or three cone theory can not explain how we, for instance, see brown, silver or gold or certain shades of colors. Additional processes must also be used to provide us with these colors. These additional processes which are purely brain processes are explained by Hering's opponent color theory. This theory is quite complex and all what is needed to be remembered is that the trichromatic (input from the different cones) and Hering's Opponent Color Theory (central color vision) theories can now basically explain our entire color vision. (For the reader interested in physics, here are the basics: Hering, a German physiologist, had noticed that we never see reddish-greens or yellowish-blues while we see yellowish- greens, blueish-reds, yellowish-reds etc. Thus, the trichromatic theory needed further additions because stimulation of red and green cones should result in reddish-green. He provided around 1900 an explanation by coupling the colors received by the brain (from the cones) into three pairs: red-green, yellow-blue and white-black. Any brain receptor that was turned off by one of these colors was then excited by its coupled color. Thus, the visual system in the brain records the differences in response of two cones to obtain the proper color sensation. Stimulation of red cones only causes red sensations, stimulation of green cones only causes green sensation but when both are stimulated at the same time they do not respond simultaneously (they are mutually exclusive) and we do not see reddish-green but we see yellow. This turns the three color process which exists in the eye into a more efficient six color process in the brain). Regardless of the exact mechanism, it is important to recognize that colors are produced and seen in the brain. This was shown in the case of the "color-blind painter". A sixty-five year old artist experienced a brain concussion and thereafter – in spite of his eyes being perfect and his cones working normally – he could not see colors and the world according to his words was like viewing the world on a black and white television. The neuronal circuits and networks in his brain which ordinarily did process and establish color vision were not functioning properly and did not color the assembled objects. Thus, certain neurons in particular areas of our brain fulfill the job of having us see the colors of the world (which of course does not have colors at all but only sends certain waves to our eyes which we then interpret as colors). Thus, the problem of color vision has been solved.

Fifth, after an object has been identified the brain must also judge the distance of this object – and place it in relation to all the other objects around it. This depth perception works in some ways similar to the formation of three dimensional objects. The most important part is our binocular vision or the use of our two eyes, in particular for near vision. Again, two very slightly different images of an object are formed on each retina which are a bit apart in our eyes. The brain can now calculate from this difference the distance of the object. This is schematically shown below:

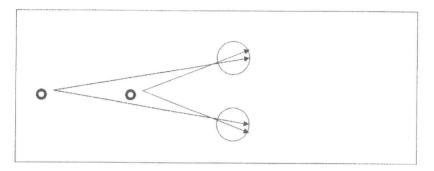

Figure 19

Also, distance plays a role in that our eyes have to move closer when viewing a near object and less so when looking into the distance. An extreme case is when an object is held very close to the eyes when they almost become cross eyed and we loose judgment if it is one or three inches away (although we know that it must be very close). Nevertheless, the brain can again calculate from the position of our eyes how far an object is from us. This is again shown schematically below:

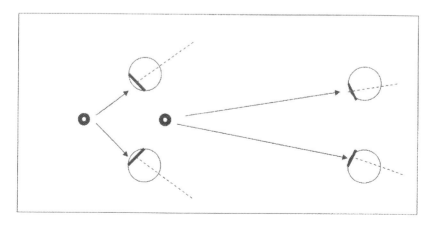

Figure 20

The importance of the two eyes can be easily demonstrated (in people using both eyes): when both eyes are open you can touch easily and quite accurately the tips of the index fingers of the left hand in front of you with one finger of the other hand. Then close one eye and do the experiment again and you will notice that you might slightly hesitate and will not be as accurate as with both eyes (you might also notice that one eye is better than the other in aligning the finger tips).

Individuals who have lost one eye have to use other ways of judging distances (some of which individuals with two functioning eyes also use). One is to judge the appearance and size of a known object. Objects are seen clearer and more detailed when close but this is lost when the objects are farther away. Objects become smaller and more blurry the farther away they are (this is a trick which painters will use to give their pictures depth perception). For instance, we know how big a car is when we stand next to it. If we now see the same car smaller we assume it must be further away. We rely on clues provided by the surroundings of an object. Parallel lines seem to merge in the distance as we all know if we look along rail road tracts (landscapers use this trick to give the impression of a "long" driveway by slightly converging their sides).

The eye also has to judge the distance between two objects. Very similar principles are used here as in the case of depth perception. Differences in the retinal images of each eye and the position of the eyes become even smaller when objects are farther and farther away from us. Thus, above facts play a major role when it comes to judging distances of objects which are close but they become less important if objects are farther away because the differences become so small that the brain cannot use them anymore. We can judge near distances pretty good but become more inaccurate as objects are farther away. Here we have to use other clues.

Occlusion helps us in that closer objects partly cover objects which are farther away. If we see a person and a second one partly covered by the first we assume that the second person must be farther away. Painters use this trick frequently to give their painting depth perception.

Although at close distance the eyes can play some tricks on. Look at the A and the B below and then move your eyes very close to them. You will see that they actually move together and touch each other:

A   B

Thus, the distance problem has been solved.

Sixth, many objects we see are in motion and we constantly have to estimate their speed. When crossing a street, the brain has to calculate the speed of an oncoming car and has to judge if it is safe to cross or not. We do this without given it much consideration (although distractions will lead to miscalculations and serious consequences). If I play baseball, I have to judge where I have to run to and how fast I have to run in order to catch a ball which has a certain speed and direction. Only skilled mathematicians could calculate my speed and direction based on above facts and it would most likely take them at least several minutes to do so. My brain – without I being aware of these mental calculations – does it all in a split second and I will perform just fine and catch the ball (at least in most cases). We all do so and even small children unaware of complicated mathematics will run at the right speed and in the right direction to catch a ball. How is this incredible feat being accomplished? As an object moves and we hold our eyes still, its image will move slowly over the retina. This allows the brain to "calculate" its speed. If the object moves and we follow it with our eyes, the eye movements allow now the brain to also "calculate" its speed. The schematic diagram shows on the left the image moving over the retina while the diagram on the right shows our eye moving from left to right:

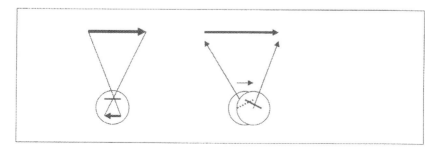

Figure 21

Up to this point, we see an object and can tell its true size, shape, color, distance and if it is moving or not. However, we still do not know what it is (it is a "naked" image without cloth).

But to emphasize again, we do not see the 'true" object but only a "copy" of this object in our brain or we never do see the world as is but only as a copy (like the copy of a true picture from the copying machine).

Sight interpretation is the next step in our visual process. Up to now we see a car but we must become aware of the image and identify and evaluate and perhaps remember what we see. This is mostly done in the associated visual areas which are located next to the visual area but are in constant communication with it.

First, the importance of the image must be evaluated and only important images are seen clearly and interpreted while unimportant images are not "seen" or suppressed (they are seen but we are not aware of them). As we drive along a busy road, we receive a lot of images – cars in front of us, buildings and trees on the roadside and perhaps birds in the air above us. Since at this time the car in front of us is most important, the eyes will focus on this car and see it distinctly while seeing but not –hopefully - paying much attention to the other objects so that we can drive safely (focusing attention, for instance, also on the birds at the same time would interfere with the visual image of the car in front of us and could lead easily to an accident and accidents do occur if our attention is diverted). This "unawareness" can sometimes become very disabling. Individuals with certain brain injuries can be blind-sighted that is they see but are not aware of what they see (see later – Ocular Problems and their Corrections and Treatments). Interference can seriously affect the formation of an image in our brain. It has been shown in human tests where two faces were shown to test subjects who could easily remember the differences between these faces. However, when the faces were shown when a light was flickering or other pictures were shown simultaneously, the subjects remembered significantly fewer differences between the faces. Subjects were shown a movie of a cocktail party and asked to follow closely a fast moving, white dressed person through the crowd of dark dressed people. Then in the middle of the picture appeared briefly a gorilla. At the end when people were asked if they saw a gorilla most said they did not see such an animal. The brain must have received the image of the gorilla but did not register it since it was unimportant for the task which was supposed to be performed. Seeing the movie a second time without paying attention to the white dressed person, people indeed saw the gorilla. Certain areas in the brain decide what is important and what is unimportant at a particular moment and make us aware of the important while suppressing the unimportant information.

Importance or meaning of the formed image derives from the image itself (it is a dog or it is a face) but also from the environment. The brain not only "sees" one object but "sees" it in conjunction with its surroundings to establish the final picture. Write a 12, 13 and 14 underneath each other (with the 1 almost touching the 2, 3, or 4) and then write an A before the 13 and a C behind it. Reading downward the 13 looks like a 13 but reading horizontally it looks like a B. Thus, the final meaning is often determined by those objects which are close by and are received at the same time.

Here, the brain can sometimes be fooled. Judging the length of both lines is affected by the short lines at their ends. The length of the upper line appears longer than that of the lower line. The length of both horizontal lines is the same. The outside lines either elongate or contract the length of the horizontal line.

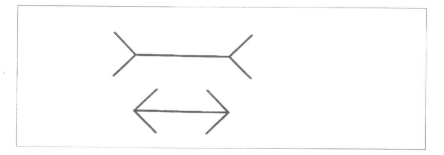

Figure 22

Second, important images must be stored and this storage can be divided into short term and long term storage. Staying at a hotel and remembering the way to the room is short term – we know it for as long as we need it and later on forget about it (again, unless something out of the ordinary did happen during this time). Long term memory stays with us for a long time or forever. We visually do remember many objects such as family members and friends, houses we lived in, interesting places we have visited, paintings which we liked and animals we have loved. But, again, very interestingly, we can remember faces the best – we can remember 100s of faces – those of our spouses, parents, children, coworkers, friends, celebrities, politicians and, perhaps, faces of people we do not like. Just imagine looking at ten paintings with similar scenes where the scenes differ slightly in shape, color and composition. How many of these ten would we remember and recognize after a few days. Not many! But faces stay with us often for a life. Interestingly, brain cells are particularly responsive to faces. We do remember different faces quite well in spite of the fact that faces are very similar in their anatomy (all have eyes, noses, cheeks, mouths) and only differ in small details (shapes of foreheads, mouths, noses, cheeks, hair and eye colors). In addition, just looking at a face we can also tell if it is a male or female face, a face belonging to a Caucasian, African or an individual of Asiatic origin and can estimate quite accurately the age of the person – again very slight changes are noticed and remembered by the brain. It has been proposed that about 400 nerve cells are necessary to recognize a face. Recent research has even claimed that a single cell in this brain area will respond to a specific face while it does not respond to other faces. We also seem to be better in identifying faces of our own ethnic group than of any other group. Caucasians have often difficulty to distinguish between faces of Asian origin and vice versa. Recently it was found that there is also a cultural component to face recognition. Western subjects would spend more time looking at the eyes and mouth of an unknown face while subjects from Asia would concentrate more on the nose. This may in part explain the custom in the western world where eye contact is preferred while it is improper in Asia. And all of this face interpretation occurs in a fraction of a second (almost simultaneously with seeing the face in the first place).

Visual memory even helps us to sometimes make sense out of nonsensical things.

Read the following two sentences:

Mnay poeple lkie sipcy deshis

or

Ynam eoeplp ekil yipcs seshid

Only the first sentence is more easily read as ""Many people like spicy dishes" because the first and last letters are correct and the brain "recognizes" the first and last letters and fills in the rest from memory. This is not the case with the second sentence where these letters are reversed.

Most people would also understand the above sentence written below with only the vowels being removed:

Mny ppl lk spc dishs

Again, the brain fills in from memory the missing vowels.

However, both short and long term memory of visual images are not infallible and can change over time either to the better or the worse. When test subjects were asked to close their eyes and to imagine a can of soda or a carton of eggs and estimate the size of each object with their hands – they overestimated the size of the object or memory made it larger than it was. Similarly, test subjects were shown a film about a car accident and a stop sign was mentioned in the ensuing discussion which actually was not seen in the movie. After this discussion, subjects were asked to recall and describe the movie. A fair number of people incorporated this stop sign into the movie and said that they actually saw a stop sign. Any lawyer can tell stories about the testimony of eye witnesses in court, who are convinced that they saw something which actually was not there or with clever cross examination can change what they have actually seen. Even things we see every day we might have trouble to remember correctly: do not look at your wrist watch and now describe the details of the watch - most people will be surprised how many details they miss although they look at the watch every day many times. But the details of the watch were not worth remembering and, thus, were not remembered.

Third, the images now will or will not arouse certain emotions. Seeing a loved one will cause a friendly feeling. Seeing a person we dislike will cause anger or hatred. A dog seen by a dog lover evokes a warm feeling while the same dog seen by a child who was bitten by a dog will cause anxiety and fear. Seeing a stranger approaching us, we quickly scan face, clothes and body posture which can signal friendly or hostile behaviors. Emotions and feelings can change to become less or more intense over time. As life continues, emotions to the same individual can often grow stronger, "mellow" or the intensity of dislike can increase to extreme hate. It has also been claimed that females can recognize emotions in a face much better than can males which would be in accordance with the general observation that females experience more emotions than do men.

To interpret the feelings of another person, again, does not need a lot of details. As a matter of fact, very few details will actually suffice and the brain will do the rest. A few distinct features of a smiling face or a sad face or a thinking face (with eyebrows raised) – depending on culture – will suffice. The following example between a happy and a sad face is just the shape of the mouth and yet happiness and sadness are immediately recognized:

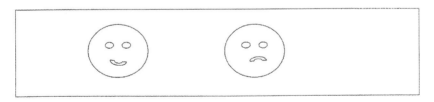

Figure 23

These details seem to be present even at a very early age. Infants were shown the smiling face repeatedly which they seem to recognize quite quickly. Then for the first time they were shown the same face but with the mouth above the eyes. Infants would look much longer at the wrong face which they recognized as unfamiliar although it had exactly the same details albeit scrambled.

And, of course, the sign language of deaf people is a prime example of how vision can make these people communicate quite effectively – and can make them work, communicate, happy, sad and wiser.

Sight projection. We now see and interpret the object or the world around us – but all these "filled in" images are still in our brains and not on the outside. Yes, the world we see, we see in our brains and we will always see and interpret what is in our brains. Thus, the brain must also have special capabilities to give us the impression that all these images are actually on the outside. This perhaps can be compared to a projector which uses the old fashion film and projects the pictures from it onto a screen. Similarly, our brain now projects all the images from our brain into the outside world and we "think" that we actually see the world as is – but no, we only see a projection of our brain's images.

That we actually only "see" in our visual cortex can be easily demonstrated as follows – we can even "see" something which is not even present. If one closes the eyes and thinks of the face of a person (e.g. mother, child) one can actually "see" this person's face although that person is not present. Also, we see faces and objects and animals during our dreams. Dreams are particularly geared to vision – we indeed "see" people, objects and animals – often in bizarre combinations and occurrences although they do not exist (but interestingly we do not seem too often to hear them speak or to smell a dirty dog or a beautiful rose). Modern brain scans have shown that the same brain areas become active (with some very slight differences) if a person sees an actual face or is asked to imagine this same face. A person suffering from a psychosis or is under the influence of hallucinogenic drugs will see people – and talk to them – although they are not there. Here, they have been produced by faulty brain processes and appear to this person as real – he or she sees them. Similarly, human experiments have shown if certain neurons and small groups of neurons are stimulated electrically (during certain brain operations where parts of the brain are exposed), then this person experiences a flash of light which might occur in a different area of the visual field depending on the neurons excited. More elaborate stimulation of larger brain areas can even produce entire pictures which do not exist in the surroundings. Thus, it is not "eye" sight but "brain" sight with which we see and experience the world around us.

<u>Sight helping systems.</u> Systems other than the visual system are also used to properly identify and "see" the images perceived. Among the many systems, let us just look at the vestibular system in our ear. This system is basically responsible for equilibrium. How could this system located in the ear then help vision? Well, draw a square and a diamond (a 45 degree tilted square) of the same size next to each other. Look at them and they appear as a square and a diamond. Tilt the paper 45 degrees and you will see the square as a diamond and the diamond as a square. Now keep the paper straight but move your head 45 degrees to one side. You will still see the original square as a square and the original diamond as a diamond. This is because the vestibular system informs the visual system that the head is tilted but the images are not – thus, the visual system corrects for this change and sees the square and diamond as they are. This is why a tree looks vertical no matter if we look straight at it or if we tilt our head to one side. This system informs the visual cortex the tree must be straight no matter how tilted our head is.

Social Interactions influencing our sight perception. Thus far, we have formed the image in our brains all by ourselves and have obtained a pretty good feeling of what we have seen. However, this image and our interpretation can often be influenced by others. Individuals were given a test where one line had to be matched to its identical counterpart among three lines drawn below. Which of the bottom lines matches the top line? About 90% of the viewers said that the left bottom line was the match (which was correct). The test subjects were then joined by other viewers who were instructed to strongly voice their opinion about the left line to be wrong and the right line to be correct. Now, about 70% of the test subjects were swayed by the opinions of others and changed their opinions. This was more obvious in younger individuals and it did diminish with age.

We do experience this phenomenon in daily life. A person with a spouse, parents or friends are looking at an object, for instance, a painting, and this person might like the painting. If others now strongly point out that this indeed is not a good painting and contains many flaws, often the first good impression of an object might change due to social influences. We might meet our new supervisor for the first time and observe a person with a kind face. Later on, this person might mistreat and disadvantage us in our job and now we will discover in his face not the kind but the malicious features. It has been said that the captain who interviewed Charles Darwin for the position of naturalist on the ship "Beagle" - who was strongly influenced by the then current theory that a particular shape of a nose would indicate a bad personality – detected such a nose in Darwin's face and was tempted not to offer him the job. Fortunately, he did change his opinion later on and nevertheless accepted Darwin on his ship. This indicates that the interpretation of what we see are not only formed within us based on our personal life experiences but can also be influenced by the opinions of others regardless if these are right or wrong.

<u>Control of ocular functions</u>. While the brain receives, identifies and interprets the images received from the eye by the optic nerves as explained above, it also sends out nerves to the eyes to control the pupils, lenses and eye movements. These effects also have to occur in both eyes simultaneously and must be synchronized. A large number of nerves leave the brain and travel to these various structures of the eye (and of course other body parts as well where they control many bodily functions and muscle movements). If it is very bright, the brain is informed about this condition and sends nerve impulses along such neurons to the iris to narrow the pupil and to do the opposite if it is getting dark. To view a near or far object, the brain sends signals along other neurons to the ciliary body to make the lens "thicker" or "thinner". To move the eyes – to look up or down, to follow a moving object or to focus on a very near or far object – the brain again controls the ocular muscles via nerve impulses traveling in still other neurons. The brain does all these functions without our control or influence – as a matter of fact we can not do these tasks voluntarily and are not even aware of them. This happens in parts of the brain which receive their input from the visual and other centers and responds accordingly.

Developmental aspects. The anatomical structures of the eye, optic nerve and brain areas develop during the growth of the child in utero and also after birth. At birth, the eyes do not dilate fully, the curvature of the lens is nearly spherical, the retina is not fully developed and the acuity is estimated to be between 20/200 and 20/400. In the next months, the eye will grow somewhat larger and the foveas will mature. However, by age one month, the baby can distinguish light and movements but ocular movements might still be uncoordinated. Between six to twelve months, acuity improves to almost normal values. The brain needs some more time for full maturation and this development is dictated by the particular genetic background or genetic blue print of the individual as well as environmental factors. Recent studies relying on vision experiments (since young infants and children cannot or not efficiently communicate) have revealed that very young infants already posses a surprising amount of brain power – a surprise to most researchers because an infant's mind had been thought to be a "tabula rasa" (blank table) or an empty brain which only acquires all the knowledge much later on in life. Nevertheless, the brain still needs time and many personal experiences and exposures to develop fully. This involves not so much plain seeing but the interpretation of what is seen by the brain and how an individual is supposed to respond. Starting with about the third month, the baby becomes aware of colors, is interested in faces and begins to associate visual stimuli with certain events. Between six to twelve months the child can now differentiate between familiar and unfamiliar people and will start to search for hidden objects – at this time a child which had lost interest in a toy when a cloth would be placed over it, will now start reaching for the toy under the cloth. Depth perception is present quite early. Infants were allowed to crawl over a table whose ends were made of transparent class. The infants would only crawl to the end of the table where the glass started but no farther. Even very young infants who could not yet crawl were uncomfortable and were crying when placed on the transparent part but not when placed on the solid part. Similarly, the protective eye reflex occurs early on in life. Infants and very young animals were placed before a screen on which a small dot was projected. Then the dot was quickly enlarged and infants and young animals all showed a quick backward reaction indicating that they were aware that "something was approaching". Infants, however, can still not distinguish between living and non-living things at this time which will be acquired only later. Six months old babies looked longer at unfamiliar pictures than familiar ones which indicates that they remember pictures quite well even at this age. Eight months old infants were shown a box which contained 80 % white and 20 % red balls – when the experimenter took four red balls and one white ball, the infants were more surprised as when he took four white and one red ball which indicates that they had – most likely subconsciously – already a feeling for proportions. Eighteen month old infants exhibited an understanding and feeling for others and to separate that person's feeling from their own. Infants observed an experimenter and two bowls of either broccoli or goldfish crackers. The experimenter ate one broccoli and acted as if he liked it and then ate one goldfish cracker and acted as if he disliked it. Then the infants were prompted to give the experimenter a piece either from the broccoli or goldfish crackers - the infants gave the broccoli (although they preferred the goldfish crackers themselves). At the age of two years, children start to recognize themselves in a mirror (few animals can do this except some apes and a few other species). This is done by placing, for instance, a spot unbeknownst on their faces and when the child looks into the mirror he or she will touch the spot. At age three years, the brain not only observes and responds but also likes to be challenged. Children were divided into two groups with each receiving the same toy – one group was shown that pressing the two levers alone or together would either raise a duck, a plane or both and the other group was only shown that when both levers were pressed both the duck and plane would be raised. The children were then given the toys to play with and those in the first group were interested in the toy only for a short time while the second group experimented with it much longer and soon discovered that individual levers would raise only one object. A three year old child if asked: what makes us think? , might answer: My brain. When asked if a dog has a brain, the child might say: yes. When asked if an ant has a brain, the child will say: no because it is too small. Similarly, if a child watches a fluid being poured into a small, bulky flask and then completely being transferred to a very tall, but narrow flask, the child would say that the tall flask contains more fluid. Similarly, if a ball of clay was flattened out on a table and the child was asked if this flattened clay was less or more than the ball, the child would say that the flattened clay was more. Thus, physical parameters such as height and size are used solely as visual measures. At age four, this changes and the child will start to conceptualize and to rationalize. Yes, the ant has a brain but it is tiny. The amounts of fluid and clay are the same in both flasks and on the table. Abstract thinking is now growing rapidly. This can be shown by the false belief test: here, children watch a person A put a marble into box X. This person then leaves the room. Now person B enters the room and places the marble into the adjacent box Y and leaves the room. Then person A re-enters the room and the children were asked in which box person A would look for the marble. Below age four, children will say Y because they know where the marble actually is. After age four, they will say box X because that is all person A knows about the whereabouts of the marble. Abstract and logical thinking develops now quite rapidly. In school, they start to perform multiple visual classification tasks and order objects in a logical sequence. Seeing the arithmetic equation:

$3+4 = 7$ the child can then write $7-4 = 3$.

After this time visual comprehension and abstract thinking continue to develop further and only at an older age begins to decline. However, the brain might develop and prefer certain proficiencies in that one person has exceptional abstract thinking skills (but cannot hammer a nail into the wall) or exceptional manual skills (but has difficulty with abstract problems). Intelligence tests usually only measure the first ability while neglecting the second one.

Individuality of vision. As outlined before, our body including the visual system is the product of our genetic material or blue print and our environment both physically as well as psychologically. Since genes and environment are unique for each individual, no two human beings will be completely alike in terms of body and personality. This means that human brains are very similar but never identical. This also means that we differ in the structure and function of our eyes and brains – sometimes only slightly and sometimes more significantly.

In case of the vision process, the function of our eyes is mostly determined by our genes and environmental influences usually cause only damaging effects such as exposure to too much sun light fostering the formation of cataracts. Most eyes among humans are very similar (except in cases of serious genetic malfunctions like the absence of certain cones resulting in color blindness). This is – as mentioned before – quite different for the brain. Again, in healthy individuals, it seems that the primary visual areas of the cortex are mostly under the influence of our genetic blue print and do not seem to show marked variations among most individuals. Most of us see the outside world quite similar. A tree or a painting or a person is seen as such by all individuals. Where the environment seems to have a greater influence than the genes is in the interpretation of what we see. A female portrait recognized by all of being that of a woman will, however, evoke very different responses. An art critic, a painter, a lay person interested in art or a person not interested in art at all, will experience and interpret the same painting quite differently depending mostly on their genetic background, education, expertise and interests. Thus, a person who sees something and interprets it differently from what I see and interpret is not "stupid" but in his or her own way is "correct" because he or she is an individual meaning a unique being with a different genetic background and environmental history.

While differences among healthy individuals exist, sick individuals will differ even more. Vision and visual interpretation among such unfortunate individuals will vary widely and it is often of no value to argue since they indeed see and interpret the world quite differently.

Thus, seeing the world is not only "brain sight" but more importantly "my brain sight" which is unique to me and can be a bit or a lot different from that of all other individuals. If this concept is appreciated it might become easier for us to understand somebody else's point of view even if it is different and perhaps seems "strange" since for this person his or her "own brain sight" is as true as is ours.

Summary. The visual processes can be divided basically into three parts including light-waves and the functions of the eyes and the brain. *Part I* is concerned with the outside world which is dark but contains invisible light-waves or electromagnetic waves which originate from the sun or artificial light sources and which are reflected from the world (people, animals, plants and objects) into our eyes. *Part II* involves the eyes. Refraction focuses these light-waves with the help of the cornea, pupil and lens onto the retina where a miniaturized but reversed picture of the objects is received. Biochemistry converts these individual waves in the millions of rods and cones into a number of chemical reactions. These reactions initiate electrical currents or nerve impulses in the adjacent nerve cells. This multitude of nerve impulses with each nerve carrying only a tiny bit of information of what is seen is then conducted by the optic nerve from each eye to the brain via the chiasm where nerve pathways partially cross. *Part III* is the brain. The brain now processes and puts together these millions of nerve inputs in various areas which, however, are in constant communication with each other (like assembling a puzzle from its individual pieces). These processes can artificially be divided as follows: <u>Sight location</u> (midbrain) involves mostly movement detection. <u>Sight recognition</u> (primary visual cortex) assembles the received individual bits and pieces into a complete image and reverses it and converts it from a two to a three dimensional image (size, shape and color). <u>Sight evaluation</u> (primary visual cortex and secondary visual areas) interprets the image and gives the image meaning such as what it is, if it is familiar or not, how far away it is, if it is moving at a given speed or not as well as evokes an emotional response and commits important information into memory. These processes produce a true "copy" of the objects seen and experienced in the brain (or better "my" brain). <u>Sight projection</u> then projects this image into the outside world where we now see light as well as where the seen object is actually located. However, it has to be remembered that we do not see the "true" world but only a "copy" of the world as formed in "my" brain.

All these processes occur in a split second – the moment I see something I can also interpret what I see. A wonder of nature and I dare to say even faster than the fastest computer.

Thus, we never see the real world but we actually only see copies of it in our brains. Since humans are individuals and differ in their genetic make-up and environments and experiences, each individual will most likely – if healthy - see the same people, animals, plants and objects a bit different and will interpret these copies often quite differently – since they exists only in the brain of the observer (influenced partly by genes but strongly by environments). Thus, it can perhaps be stated that each person experiences only "his/her own personal world" or the world is seen and experienced in "his or her brain". This should teach us tolerance because my brain is slightly different from the brains of other people and, thus, experiencing "my world" might sometimes be different from that of other people – although their world is equally true for them.

Ocular Problems and their Corrections and Treatments

Introduction. Fortunately, the majority of people have either healthy eyes and proper vision or experience only minor ocular problems which can relatively easily be cured or corrected. Unfortunately, some suffer from severe ocular problems which can nevertheless be partially corrected or treated today while some individuals can regrettably not be helped at all at this time.

Problems with our eyes which we encounter can perhaps be divided into problems which occur normally during aging, are inborn and/or are encountered during our life like injuries or infections. This chapter will discuss some of the major optical and medical problems encountered more frequently with an overview of their respective optical, medical and surgical treatments if available. It will not discuss serious problems like major trauma or injuries to the eye, cancer, certain major brain disorders or immunological problems. These are strictly matters for the health professions. It must also be added that this chapter is not intended to serve as a medical guide for self-- treatment or self-medication but more to identify and recognize problems before they become serious or untreatable. Visual and medical problems of the eye depending on their nature must only be dealt with by a licensed health professional such as a physician, ophthalmologist, optometrist or optician.

Most individuals are born with a healthy visual system or a system which shows only minor health problems (severe problems will be discussed later) and their eyes and brain function well within healthy limits. As the body ages, detrimental changes occur (perhaps by a wear and tear process) including the eyes and brain. However, it is well known that people age differently and that there is a significant difference between chronological and biological age. A seventy year old person can have the physique of a fifty year old and a fifty year old can be biologically seventy years old. This aging process and our death depend largely on our inherited genes (not just from parents but also grand parents and great grand parents – since genetic traits can skip one or more generations) and family history is a good predictor of our aging process (as it is to other biological and medical conditions as well). This of course excludes accidents and adverse natural courses. Apparently, our DNA has an intrinsic program which tells our cells how many times they can divide and when to stop dividing and die. Our genes not only make us alive but also cause an end to our lives. This has been shown experimentally in that cells from people of different ages were obtained and then grown in Petri dishes in the laboratory where they would divide and multiply. Cells from young people would divide many times before they would stop and die. Cells from middle aged people would show only half the divisions before death would occur and cells from old people would only divide twice or three times before they would die. Our genes determine our life span. However, our lifestyle can also significantly slow down or speed up the way we grow old. Exercise, proper nutrition, sufficient sleep and a healthy outlook seem to prolong while inactivity, overweight, excessive sun exposure, poor dietary habits, excessive alcohol use or smoking can shorten our lives. Problems which occur early on in life or become very severe during our lives are usually genetically in origin (again, not considering accidental injuries to the eyes or brain damage caused by trauma).

Optical properties of the eye. One of the most frequently encountered visual problems fall in to the realm of optics or problems with seeing clearly and accurately either near or far or both. They are caused by improper refraction and are mostly the result of imperfections of the length of the eye, the cornea and/or lens. In the healthy eye, the light rays are focused via cornea, pupil and lens directly on the retina which are all in perfect alignment to assure the production of a clear image on the latter. In some individuals the eye ball can be too short or too long and the refracted light waves meet and focus the image either behind or before the retina. This can occur at a young age and some of these individuals will "outgrow" this problem as the eye changes during normal growth. However, many others – in particularly those with a family history of vision problems – will not. This indicates that it is a genetic or inborn problem. If the eye remains too long or the cornea is too curved, the images form before the retina. This is referred to as near-sightedness or myopia because the individual can see close objects clearly but sees objects farther away as blurry. If the eye remains too short or the cornea is too flat, light rays focus behind the retina. This is referred to as far-sightedness or hyperopia also named hypermetropia because the individual can see far but cannot see clearly close objects. If the cornea or lens do not have a smooth curvature but show slight deviations, light rays focus on different points of the retina and result in distorted vision. This is referred to as astigmatism. If the lens loses flexibility and becomes rigid – usually at an older age – it fails to accommodate to near distances. Such individuals can see well in the distance but cannot read fine print or have to move the reading material farther away from the eyes in order to see it more clearly. This is called presbyopia.

Vision is measured in relative numbers. A vision of 20/20 means that a person can stand 20 feet away from the eye chart and can see what a "normal" individual (or most people with healthy eyes) can see. In metric terms, the standard is 6 meters and it is then called 6/6 vision. A person with 20/40 vision must be 20 feet away from the eye chart in order to see what individuals with normal vision can see at a distance of 40 feet. Thus, this is a relative measure based on what the majority of people with "normal" vision can see.

Most of these problems – unless very severe – can easily be corrected. In most instances eyeglasses or contact lenses will be prescribed which will bend or refract incoming light rays so that they meet more properly on the retina. They use lenses which can be convex which concentrates light in one point (called the focal point) or can be concave which diverge light.

The power of a convex lens or its curvature is measured in terms of diopters (a diopter is equal to the reciprocal of the focal length measured in meters or a 3-diopter lens brings parallel rays of light to a focal point at one third of a meter – 1 m divided by 3 equals one third m). The human eye has about a power of 60 diopters or it focuses parallel rays arriving at the cornea at a distance of about 17 mm behind the cornea which is exactly the location of the retina (1 m divided by 60 equals 0.017 m or 17 mm). The power of a concave lens is measured in negative diopters (or the focal point is before the lens).

Old fashioned eye glasses are worn on the nose. Contact lenses are worn directly on the eye. Contact lenses are strict prescription items and must be properly fitted by an ophthalmologist or optometrist. They consist of different materials such as the most often used soft lenses which are made from a gel-like, water-containing plastic and the "oxygen permeable" lenses which are made from rigid, waterless plastics. The latter are particularly good for eyes with high astigmatism. Recently, new silicon hydrogel contact lenses have become the contact lenses of choice because they allow more oxygen to pass through the contact lens to the cornea and they are less prone to dehydration. Until 1979, everyone who wore contact lenses removed and cleaned them nightly. The introduction of "extended wear" lenses enabled wearers to sleep with their contacts. Lenses are now classified into daily wear (must be removed nightly), extended wear (can be worn usually for seven days consecutively without removal during the night) and continuous wear lenses (can be worn for 30 consecutive nights).

Contact lens wearers – and there are about 30 million in the United States – are exposed to some health risks some of which are caused by individualized responses (that is not all eyes respond equally to contact lenses) or are self-inflicted (caused by negligence or poor hygiene). If contact lenses are ill-fitted or changes in the tear film occur, the individual experiences discomfort and red eyes usually after wearing these lenses for some time. The solution might be refitting of the lenses. Some individuals develop a giant papillary conjunctivitis which manifests itself as red, itchy eyes and sometimes includes poor vision. It is caused by the formation of large or giant papillae (nipple-shaped growths) under the eyelids. It is an immune reaction unique to these individuals. Treatment generally requires discontinuance of or in milder cases time limitation of the use of contact lenses. Sometimes, drug treatment is required. Proteins and lipids – with soft lenses mostly - can deposit on the lenses causing discomfort and itching. They also can serve as breeding grounds for bacteria. In most cases, a new lens is required and good enzymatic cleaning might solve this problem. Hypersensitivity reactions to contact lens solutions are also encountered and individuals experience red, irritated eyes and difficulty in wearing the contact lenses. In many cases, this reaction occurs in response to the cleaning solutions and the use of a solution with a different preservative is all that is required. Hard, rigid, gas-permeable or sometimes soft contact lenses can lead to changes in the curvature of the cornea and the individual notices a worsening of vision over time. The treatment is discontinuance of the use of contact lenses until the cornea stabilizes and refitting of new lenses. Infections caused by contact lenses will be discussed later. Most of the problems caused by contact lenses can be attributed to over-wear or improper wear of contact lenses, poor lens hygiene, individual sensitivity to lens materials and solutions and/or a poor contact lens fit.

Shown below are ways how lenses correct two vision problems. In the hyperopic eye the proper convex lens bundles the light rays so that they converge sooner or right at the retina. In the myopic eye the proper concave lens diverges the light rays farther on or again right at the retina. Thus, the ophthalmologist or optometrist will have to try different lenses until that lens will be found which will focus the light rays right onto the retina.

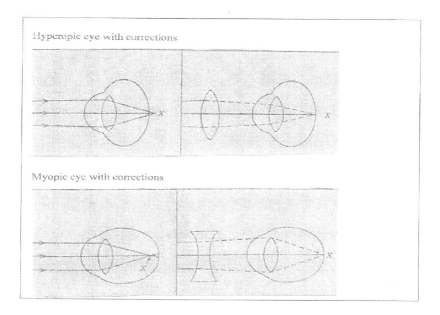

Figure 24

In addition to eyeglasses and contact lenses, surgery can be performed to correct these vision problems. One of these procedures is LASIK (Laser-Assisted in situ Keratomileusis) treatment. This procedure is estimated to be performed about 1 million times per year in the USA. It is based on changing the highly refractive power of the cornea. A special device creates a thin corneal flap which is laid aside. Then a laser sculpts the patient's eyeglass prescription onto the cornea by removing a layer of the cornea to produce a predetermined curvature. The corneal flap is then placed back on the cornea where it will attach itself over the next days. This is done on an outpatient basis.

The procedure corrects vision problems such as myopia, hyperopia and astigmatism but not presbyopia (which is a problem of the lens). Most people choose to have their myopic condition corrected but will have to use reading glasses later on in life. The satisfaction rate is high and estimated to be well over 90%. Complications are relatively rare and depend on the skill of the ophthalmologist and the response of an individual eye. Estimates of problems are less than 5 % and range from unsatisfactory correction (sometimes requiring another procedure) over experience of a glare and dry eye to impaired –and very rarely – lost vision. Caucasian eyes have been found to tolerate this procedure better than Asiatic eyes. It has also been estimated that the use of contact lenses carries a higher risk of adverse effects than LASIK. Another laser procedure is called PRK (photorefractive Keratectomy). This procedure does not create a corneal flap like LASIK but reshapes the cornea directly so that the cornea's structural integrity is affected less. It is used mostly for individuals with specially shaped corneas where LASIK might not be indicated and seems to produce fewer side effects.

Lids. During aging, the lids can lose hair and this loss might reduce light protection from the upper lids. Fortunately, a drug has been recently discovered which can re-grow some of the lost hair (this capability was actually discovered from an unexpected side effect of the drug which was used for the treatment of glaucoma). Another common eyelid problem involves the development of an age-related baggy upper lid which can also restrict the visual field and surgery can now easily correct this problem. Infections are described later.

Tear film. This aqueous film composed of water, lipids, nutrients and immune components is constantly produced by the glands to keep the eye moist. Part of it evaporates and part drains though channels located along the inner part of the eyes into the nasal cavity. This film has to be constantly renewed. At older ages, this production can slow down or the composition of the tear film can change and – some mostly older - individuals will experience an uncomfortable "dry" eye (which does not mean the eye is indeed dry but the tear film is not sufficiently thick or splits and shows dry areas). This decrease in the ocular "lubricant" does not only cause discomfort but can also be damaging to the eye. In addition, certain medications (some anticholinergic, antihistaminic, antidepressant or antipsychotic drugs) are known to decrease tear formation as well as certain diseases such as rheumatoid arthritis, lupus and sarcoidosis (an accumulation of inflammatory cells forming nodules in tissues). A dry eye manifests itself as a stinging, burning or scratchy sensation in your eyes, stringy mucus in or around your eyes, eye fatigue after short periods of reading, sensitivity to light, difficulty wearing contact lenses and blurred vision, often becoming worse at the end of the day or after visually focusing for a prolonged period of time on a nearby tasks. Paradoxically, the eyes might also water excessively because changes in the tear film can stimulate certain glands to go into over-production. Both eyes are usually affected. Depending on the onset, duration and severity of this problem, an eye examination is usually indicated to rule out more serious causes. If the cause is a certain medication then it might only be temporary until the drug is not needed any longer or the drug can be switched to another which affects the eyes less. In most cases it is harmless and "artificial tears" might solve this problem. A variety of non-prescription medications are available. These tear fluids are manufactured to come close to the composition of the natural tear film so that they can substitute for the natural tear film without causing discomfort. In severe cases where "artificial tears" do not help prescription drugs can be used or plugs can be inserted into the drainage channels of the eyes to prevent drainage and keep natural and artificial tears longer on top of the eye.

Cornea. Next, the cornea will slowly become a bit cloudy over the years which will cause some glare by light scattering and decrease contrast but will usually not present a major problem unless the cornea had endured previously serious infections or injuries with scars which could make vision blurry. Many older individuals will show the "arcus senilis" or a ring visible around the cornea. This produces a minor loss of peripheral vision which is harmless and usually not noticed by the individual. This ring is usually not associated with high cholesterol levels.

Extremely high cholesterol and triglyceride levels are sometimes, but not usually, associated with a similar gray or white arc visible around the entire cornea in younger adults. Again no major visual impairment is noticed. As the cornea ages it also becomes more susceptible to infections.

The cells lining the back of the cornea are called the "endothelium". They can start dying off over time. If this process is accelerated, the condition is called Fuch's disease or endothelial dystrophy. Since these cells pump the water out of the cornea, the cornea fills up with water and swells and vision becomes blurry. Sometimes the water builds up inside so much that painful corneal blisters can form. At first, such a person will awaken with blurred vision that will gradually clear during the day. As the disease worsens, this swelling will remain constant and reduce vision throughout the day. Treatment includes topical hypertonic saline and the use of a hairdryer to dehydrate the superficial corneal layers, therapeutic soft contact lenses and finally a corneal transplant might be needed.

Iris. The iris or the visible colored portion of the eye will slowly lose elasticity which results in a decreased ability to narrow the pupil. An insufficiently contracted pupil can cause excessive glare on sunny days and individuals will experience some photophobia or intolerance of light. A more serious problem can arise when the aging iris starts to shed pigments which can lodge in the trabecular meshwork (through which the ocular fluid drains) and interfere with the outflow of the intraocular fluid. This can increase intraocular pressure (called open angle glaucoma) which untreated can lead to loss of vision. Fortunately, treatments are available (see below).

Lens. The lens which is suspended by ligaments in the ciliary body also loses elasticity over time, fails to contract properly and does not allow for proper focusing. This can be corrected with glasses. The lens might become yellow which would interfere with color vision in particular the true perception of blue. Elderly ladies might dye their white hair slightly blue but with the impairment through a yellowish lens will overdue it and their hair looks to us – not to them – very blue.

More serious is the formation of cloudy spots in one or more areas within the lens or cataracts which prevent light from reaching the retina. The word cataract is derived from the Latin word for "waterfall" since it was believed that a fluid from the brain would flow over the lens and solidify preventing the lens from "seeing" (the lens was thought at this time to be the site of vision). This cloudiness can be caused by clumping of lenticular proteins and/or their breakdowns into yellowish-brownish pigments. These problems can occur in the middle of the lens (nuclear cataracts) or on its outsides (cortical cataracts) as well as in the back near the capsule (posterior subcapsular cataracts).

Cataracts develop usually at an older age which must not mean that everybody will develop cataracts. Risk factors include genetic predispositions (family history), exposure to too much sunlight, cigarette smoking, eye injuries, obesity, extensive exposure to radiation, certain illnesses like diabetes and drugs like corticosteroids. Cataracts are painless but can cause a number of vision problems like cloudy and blurry vision, glares and halos, faded colors and sometimes double vision. If untreated they lead to blindness (which is still a significant problem in undeveloped countries). Little can be done to prevent cataract formation except reducing above risk factors if possible. The use of vitamins and antioxidants – widely promoted – has not been scientifically found to be effective.

Fortunately, cataracts can be treated readily, effectively and safely today. These treatments involve removal of the natural lens and implantation of an artificial lens. There are several possible operations available but the most common is the phacoemulsification. It can be performed under local anesthesia (awake) or general anesthesia (unconscious) on an outpatient basis. The actual procedure takes about 5 minutes with more time spent pre- and post-operatively. No pain will be experienced and the patient might only see some bright lights and colors during surgery. The ophthalmologist using a microscope will make a tiny opening in the outer edge of the cornea (about 3 mm), insert first an instrument to remove the front of the capsule and then a probe emitting ultrasound waves which break the lens into very fine fragments which will be vacuumed out of the eye. Then the artificial lens is inserted. After the operation the tiny incision closes by itself and the patient should only wear a perforated plastic patch at night to prevent any accidental poking of a finger into the eye.

In some cases extracapsular surgery is performed with a longer incision on the side of the cornea and removing the cloudy core of the lens in one piece. The rest of the lens is removed by suction and the artificial lens is inserted.

There are several intraocular lenses or IOLs available. One type is shown below:

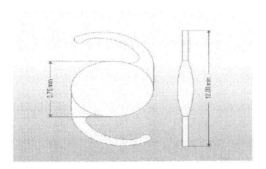

Figure 25

The proper lens is selected based on the optical measurements of the eye taken before the lens implantation and based on the wishes of the patient. A "monofocal lens" can be used which will provide either far or near vision. If they are implanted into both eyes, the patient then only needs reading glasses if a lens for distant vision had been selected. However, a lens for near vision can be implanted into one eye and one for far vision into the other eye and the patient would not need glasses at all. Recently, accommodating lenses have been invented. Such a lens can curve and flex just like our natural lens and the patient can see either near or far. After surgery, the use of an anti-inflammatory drug and an antibiotic are recommended. In rare cases, IOLs can not be used and the patient's vision is then corrected with eye glasses or contact lenses.

Cataract surgery is a very routine procedure today and about three million surgeries are performed in the USA per year. Complications after cataract surgery are extremely rare and most can be treated successfully. They include inflammation, infection, bleeding, swelling, retinal detachment and glaucoma. In some cases the lens might shift which either causes minor problems or additional surgery can bring the lens back into place. These risks increase for people who have other eye diseases or serious medical problems.

Ophthalmologists also recommend having the natural lens removed as a person gets older even if he or she has no significant lens clouding or vision problems. This recommendation is a preventive measure since the lens can become eventually so hard and difficult to emulsify if a cataract operation would be necessary later on. If the lens is too hard, removal will be more complicated and difficult and can give rise to unwanted complications.

One complication which occurs in a fair number of patients is post surgical clouding of vision. This is caused in that the posterior part of the capsule becomes cloudy. This is easily treated with a YAG (yttrium-aluminum-garnet) laser. Here, the ophthalmologist – without anesthesia and within 1 minute – opens a hole in the back of the capsule so that light will again fall unhindered onto the retina.

Vitreous. An annoying problem is the appearance of "floaters" in the eye. As the vitreous degenerates, microscopic fibers within it tend to clump together and start to shift around as the eye moves casting tiny shadows on the retina, which are seen as eye floaters. They are perceived as little "objects" or "insects" flying before the eye. In most cases (except in some instances when signaling a retinal detachment) they are annoying but harmless and individuals will adapt to them (while in the beginning they might try to chase the "insect" away while later on these floaters will be generally ignored).

Retina. Various problems can occur with the retina during aging. The photosensitive cells in the macula and in particular its most central part the fovea become damaged and die resulting in "age-related macular degeneration" or AMD. This results in a loss of acute central vision which becomes blurred while peripheral vision remains relatively intact. Causes of this problem include genetic predispositions, age, cigarette smoking, obesity, high blood pressure and elevated levels of c-reactive protein (a marker of inflammations in the body). Symptoms of AMD include blurred vision, straight lines appear to have a kink, blank spots in central vision and colors become dimmer.

There are two forms of AMD. One is called the non-neovascular or "dry" form. It is characterized by shrinkage of macular tissue and the formation of drusen (debris under the retina). It progresses very slowly and might stabilize intermittently. Vision is usually not seriously impaired in most individuals but will eventually progress to serious vision loss. About 90% of individuals with AMD have this type. The other type is called neovascular or "wet" AMD. It arises from the dry form and is caused by the sprouting of new blood vessels in the eye. These vessels will start to leak blood and fluid and cause scar tissue formation which replaces the photosensitive cells in the macula. This can occur quite quickly, is much more dangerous and requires immediate medical attention.

Older eyes require more thorough and frequent eye examinations. The chance of developing AMD can now be predicted based on a score developed by ophthalmologists. If the ophthalmologist or optometrist detects certain changes they assign a score ranging from 1- 4. A patient with a score of 1 has a 3% chance and a patient with a score of 4 has a 50% chance of developing AMD within the next 5 years.

AMD cannot be prevented or cured but progression of an existing "dry" AMD can be slowed and the harmful effects of a "wet" AMD can be minimized. Recently, use of a combination of vitamins, a mineral and a certain organic compound (vitamins A, C and E, zinc and lutein) has been shown not to prevent but to somewhat slow the progression of the "dry" form. The "wet" form can be treated by retinal specialists by destroying the newly formed, harmful blood vessel through various techniques involving either certain drugs or a combination of a drug and a laser. Injection of certain dyes can help the ophthalmologist to identify the new and leaky blood vessels and laser application can destroy these vessels selectively (this is called photocoagulation). Another procedure involves injection of a drug (verteporfin) which binds preferentially to newly formed blood vessels and in conjunction with a laser application closes these vessels. Pure drug therapy involves use of drugs which interfere with the formation of new blood vessels. For a blood vessel to form, a protein called vascular endothelial growth factor (VEGF) is necessary. Drugs (pegaptanib and ranibizumab) can inhibit the action of VEGF and prevent formation of new vessels. These drugs seem to be more effective than the laser therapies but are unfortunately very expensive. All these treatments have been found to prevent the harmful effects of the "wet" form and to preserve vision.

In addition, research has shown that people with AMD have quick and constantly shifting eye movements which may make poor vision even worse. Studies suggest teaching these individuals to use longer and slower scanning movements of the environment which might help to increase visual comprehension. Magnification devices can also be helpful.

Another problem is retinal detachment. Retinal detachment occurs when parts of the inner layer of the retina detach from their background. It often begins when the vitreous shrinks and separates from the retina. In most cases, vitreous separation occurs as one ages and is usually harmless. Sometimes though, it can tear the retina. This happens when the vitreous gel is strongly attached to the retina. In this case, it pulls so hard that the retina tears. The tear allows fluid to collect behind the retina and may cause the retina to detach more and more from its background loosing eventually its oxygen and nutrient supply. Ultimately, these cells die and vision is lost.

Also, eye injuries and trauma (such as in boxers who have experienced frequent blows to the eyes) and diseases like diabetes can cause problems. Warning signals are flashes of light, lightning streaks, dark shadows across part of the visual field or a sudden loss of peripheral vision that gets worse over time. These signs require immediate medical help since untreated significant loss of vision or blindness can result. There are different procedures available today to help and to prevent vision loss. These procedures are often performed to close the tear so that the retina can attach itself again to the background. These treatments use lasers or a freezing probe to seal the tear in the retina. Other procedures employ the use of gases injected into the eye to force the detached retina back onto the back of the eye. Devices applied to the outer eye (scleral buckling) try to contract the eye and to force the detached retina back to its original place. Most of these procedures are performed on an outpatient basis.

Blood vessels in the eye supply the retina with oxygen and nutrients. Any interference with blood flow may cause problems and can sometimes lead to transient loss of vision referred to as amaurosis fugax. Patients describe it as a transient monocular vision loss like a curtain coming down vertically or blindness, dimming, fogging or blurring. It typically lasts only a few seconds, but can last minutes or even hours. This can be caused by a variety of causes like a brief vascular spasm (constriction) of the blood vessels or a blood clot getting temporarily stuck mostly in atherosclerotic vessels (hardened blood vessels with cholesterol deposits narrowing the passage way). Such an occurrence must be brought to the attention of an ophthalmologist immediately.

Optic nerve. The optic nerve loses its speed with which it conducts nerve impulses from the retina to the individual brain areas during aging. At age 70, a 25 % decrease in this conductance speed can be assumed. Thus, the time to see an object in the brain will be slightly, for many hardly noticeable, delayed. This manifests itself in decreased visual reflexes which can become dangerous, for instance, when driving a car. The optic nerve can also get inflamed (optic neuritis) and the patient might experience a sudden foggy, blurry vision or loss of vision, pain by movement of the affected eye and loss of some color vision. The condition might heal by itself or medications can be used (like steroids or immunosuppressant drugs) to speed up the healing process.

Glaucoma. Problems can arise with the intraocular pressure (IOP). The fluid in the eye is produced by the ciliary processes, flows through the pupil and leaves through the trabecular meshwork. Inflow and outflow result in the IOP which keeps the eye from collapsing. The channels of the trabecular meshwork are very sensitive to changes in this pressure (the eye is an enclosed chamber). If the pressure increases, the channels open, allow more outflow and decrease the pressure. If the pressure falls, the channels close, decrease the outflow and the pressure inside the eye rises. Due to this mechanism the pressure is kept within certain limits just right for the eye to function normally. It is easily measured with a tonometer. There are different types like the tonometer which uses a probe to gently flatten part of your cornea. The force needed to flatten your cornea is a measure of the pressure inside the eye.

There is also a tonometer which uses an air puff to measure the ocular pressure. A normal pressure is considered to be between 10 to 20 mm. However, if the pressure in the eyes increases the retina and the optic nerve will be damaged leading to vision impairment and eventually blindness. An increased IOP is referred to as glaucoma although visual loss is actually due to the damage of the retina and optic nerve. The increase in IOP is only one indication but careful visual field (perimetry) and eye examinations by an ophthalmologist or optometrist are required to actually make the final diagnosis, decide on treatment options and to determine the success of any treatment.

There are different types of glaucoma. Only the two most common of these conditions will be described in more detail below.

The first is called the primary open angle glaucoma. It affects about 2-3 million individuals in the USA. The problem is with the trabecular meshwork which drains insufficiently and causes the IOP to increase. This problem can have various reasons such as blockage by shedded pigments from the iris and other as yet unknown causes. It has a genetic background, occurs often in individuals with very thin corneas, is more common in Blacks and Hispanics and can be caused by certain drugs like the corticosteroids. The damage to the eyes is slowly progressing with a loss of peripheral vision first which is often unnoticed by the individual in the beginning since there is no discomfort, pain or any other signs. Later on, the visual field will become smaller (tunnel vision) and if not treated blindness might ensue. In some cases, even what is considered a normal pressure can be too high for a particular eye and can result in optic nerve damage (this is called low tension glaucoma). It requires the same treatment.

There are various treatments available which will not cure but slow down or arrest the progression of damage and preserve vision. A large number of different drugs can be applied to the eye which can either decrease inflow or increase outflow and restore normal pressure. These different drugs are called beta blockers, selective alpha receptor agonists, carbonic anhydrase inhibitors, prostaglandin analogues, sympathomimetics and miotics. Due to this large selection of drugs, the right drug for the right patient can be easily found which means that the therapeutic effects can be optimized and the adverse reactions can be minimized. Most patients tolerate these medications well. In many cases, a combination of drugs might become necessary during therapy. For those who do not benefit from medications (about 10%) surgical procedures become necessary. They are performed in most cases by using local anesthesia and are quite safe. Laser trabecular surgery burns a tiny hole into the trabecular meshwork which increases outflow. Filtration surgery opens mechanically a passage through the meshwork for better drainage. After this, either no medications or some medications might be necessary depending on the patient. Rarely, shunts have to be implanted through the eye to drain the intraocular fluid or the ciliary body as a source of fluid production has to be destroyed. These measures drastically slow down damage to the optic nerve and can preserve vision for a very long time.

It has been widely asserted that marihuana smoking has a significant eye pressure lowering effect. This is indeed the case in that the smoke of cannabis contains a number of compounds which do lower intraocular pressure. These compounds were not effective when applied topically. However, prescription medications which can be applied topically are more effective without showing some of the unwanted effects of marihuana smoke on the body and brain.

The second type is called acute angle-closure glaucoma. Here, predisposed individuals have a shallow that is narrower angle between the iris and cornea than normal individuals. Usually, this presents no problem and the drainage remains efficient. However, if the iris retracts (the pupil now becomes large), the iris starts to "crowd' the angle, reduce outflow and finally stop outflow all together. This can be precipitated by some medications (but only in individuals with such a narrow angle while people with a normal angle remain unaffected) or other conditions. In this case, the pressure inside the eye rises quickly very high and the patient experiences nausea and pain. If untreated, this type of glaucoma can cause blindness in a few days. This is a medical emergency and medical help must be sought as soon as possible. If treated with medications first and then with ocular surgery, vision can be preserved and similar attacks can be prevented in the future.

Environmental influences. Additional problems can arise from our environment. They can be of different origins and severities. Trauma to the eye can cause minor, reversible problems which can be taken care of by an ophthalmologist. However, severe accidents can lead to major, irreversible damage or can even result in blindness. Irritating chemicals, allergens and microbes can lead to eye irritations, inflammations, allergic reactions and infections. Here, the genetic disposition of the individual will often play a significant role in that some individuals are more while others are less affected by these environmental factors. Some of these problems are listed below.

Inflammation. An inflammation is generally a protective and helpful immune response of the body to protect, prevent and repair damage to our bodily tissues. It consists of changes in blood flow, an increase in permeability of blood vessels, and the migration of fluid, proteins, and white blood cells from the blood to the site of a tissue which has been damaged or infected. The cardinal signs of an inflammation are redness, warmth, swelling and pain. It can be caused by microorganisms, physical trauma, chemicals, after surgeries and unknown causes. A short term inflammatory response is called acute inflammation, while a long term response is called chronic inflammation. An inflammation is classified by the tissue affected and the suffix –itis. If the conjunctiva is affected it is referred to as conjunctivitis. In addition, the causes of the inflammation are mentioned. A bacterial caused inflammation is a bacterial conjunctivitis, an allergic inflammation is an allergic conjunctivitis and so forth. As mentioned before, the inflammatory response is a beneficial reaction of the body. However, if such an inflammation over-reacts and becomes excessive, it can damage the eye. Sometimes, an inflammation can be caused by the body's own immune system. It is then called an autoimmune disease. In these cases, inflammations must be suppressed by drugs to prevent damage to the eye.

A potentially serious problem arises if the macula becomes inflamed or a macular edema occurs. This is a swelling or thickening of the macula, it is painless and can lead to blurred or distorted vision and if not treated to blindness. It can occur after cataract surgery, age-related macular degeneration (ARMD), eye injury, diabetes, retinal vein occlusion or in response to certain drug treatments. If it occurs after surgery, it is usually reversible. The condition can be treated and responds well in most cases to topical steroids such as dexamethasone or prednisolone and drugs called NSAIDs such as ketorolac or bromfenac. In severe cases, a steroid injection is given behind the eye (retrobulbar). A recent treatment involves the application of a steroid depository behind the eye which insures a long and constant flow of the anti-inflammatory drug.

Allergy. The allergic reaction is highly individualized in that some substances in our environment (pollen, dust, animal dandruff, cosmetics, certain drugs and other substances which are called allergens) cause in some, but not all, individuals an immune system response referred to as an allergic reaction. Family history is a pretty good indicator if you will be affected by certain allergens. It is estimated that about 50 million Americans suffer from this misery which is not dangerous but highly discomforting and annoying. This allergic reaction can be caused by tiny amounts of an allergen like a few pollen, the injection of a minuscule quantity of a bee's venom or the mere smell of shrimp. It can occur all over the body (hives) but in the eye it manifests itself mostly in the conjunctiva with watery (resulting in blurred vision), red, burning and itchy eyes. The allergic reactions can occur only at particular times of the year (seasonal allergies) or year round (perennial allergies). The clinical signs can occur right after exposure (called an immediate allergic or type I reaction) or after 1 -2 days only (called a delayed allergic or type IV allergic reaction). Biologically and medically both reactions differ in that type I reactions are caused by a substance in the body called IgE and histamine whereas the type IV reaction is caused by certain immune cells called T-cells. The type I can escalate into an anaphylactic shock where the individual can die due to extremely low blood pressure and bronchoconstriction (here the Epipen – a portable injection device containing adrenalin or epinephrine - can help and keep this individual alive until the emergency room can intervene). The best way to avoid or terminate such reactions is to identify and to avoid the allergen. This is often easier in case of a type I reaction which occurs shortly after exposure (during a visit in a house with a cat the eyes start to become itchy and watery; here the cat is the most likely cause) but more difficult in the case of a type IV reaction where 2 or more days may pass between exposure and the occurrence of clinical signs. Many cosmetic induced reactions fall into this latter category (the cosmetic might be tried the day before but not on the day the eyes start to show an allergic reaction; most individuals might not think of something which occurred 1 or 2 days earlier as the causative agent). If the allergen can not be identified or can not be avoided (like pollen in the air), medications are available which are applied to the eye. They can be prescribed after an eye examination (to rule out other problems) by an ophthalmologist or, in some states, by an optometrist. They are quite effective and relatively safe. Medications might differ depending on the presence of a type I or IV reaction. In the case of type I reactions, mast cell stabilizers can be prescribed prophylactically (before onset of the reaction) to prevent its occurrence or topical antihistamines or steroids. In additions, systemic antihistamines (taken orally) and other topical (applied to the eye) medications such as decongestions (blood vessel constrictors) can be used. In case of a type IV reaction, steroids are usually the drugs of choice. If taken as prescribed they are effective and relatively safe.

Infections. Infections of the eye are another problem which can range from mild to severe. They are caused by bacteria, viruses, fungi or amoeba. Usually, the tear film contains many of these microbes but the eye has a strong defense system against them. Sometimes the immune defenses are overwhelmed and microbial infections occur. Most eye infections are bacterial in nature while viral and fungal infections are rarer and often occur in people with a compromised immune system such as transplant patients (where the immune system is medically weakened to prevent organ rejection), AIDS patients (where the virus affects and impairs the immune system) or after eye injuries (where the microbes have easy access into the inner parts of the eye). They can affect all parts of the eye including the lids. Some specific infections are listed below.

Bacterial infections will be discussed first. Bacteria are one cell organisms which multiply – in or outside the body- through cell divisions. It has been estimated that one bacterium in the eye can multiply and produce 1 million new bacteria in one day. They consist basically of a cell wall (not found in human cells which have only a cell membrane), a DNA accumulation in the cell (no nucleus as is found in human cells) and protoplasm containing various substances and enzymes. Bacteria occur in many different forms, shapes and sizes. They are classified as different species as well as strains and sub-strains. They can also be divided into good or benign (causing no harm or are even helpful to the body) and harmful or pathogenic (causing harm to the body). The human body houses more bacteria than it has cells and they number in the trillions. Most of the times, they do not produce a health problem because the immune system as well as the benign bacteria keep the pathogenic ones in check. Sometimes pathogenic bacteria overwhelm this defense system, multiply and cause an infection. Each pathogenic species or strain causes a specific effect on the body or a particular infection or disease. They often manifest themselves as an inflammation (redness, swelling, pain), fever and the formation of yellowish/greenish pus (consisting mostly of killed white blood cells). The identification of such bacteria causing a special problem is crucial for the selection of the right anti-bacterial medications.

Infections which affect the eye can be local events or can sometimes arise from systemic diseases. A sty (hordeolum) results from an infection of a particular gland or hair follicle of the eye lid. It develops at the basis of the lid. The eye feels irritated and a small yellowish spot appears. Treatment consists of warm compresses and it will disappear in about ten days. If the inflammation is inside the lid, it is called a chalazion. Symptoms are usually more severe and include eye lid swelling and treatment might include antibiotics and corticosteroids. They usually disappear in about a few months.

Blepharitis is a more generalized inflamed eyelid. The eyes might feel gritty, tired and are sensitive to light. Treatment consists of artificial tears, eye lid cleansing and in more severe cases antibiotics and/or corticosteroids. An infection of the conjunctiva is called "pink eye" (conjunctivitis) which is very contagious but usually benign. It manifests itself as eye redness, eye pain and light sensitivity. It will usually heal by itself but sometimes might require medications like antibiotics (redness in the eye can also be caused by an allergy or a viral infection). One of the most dreaded complications of contact lens wear is a corneal ulcer caused by a bacterial infection. The condition manifests itself as a red, painful eye with pus discharge, and perhaps impaired vision. The use of antibiotics resolves this problem in most cases– unfortunately, not in all. Infections of the inner eye are more serious and require intense medical care. However, based on a thorough eye examination, the clinical signs and sometimes laboratory tests, an ophthalmologist can usually make a good diagnosis and can chose the right antibiotic. There is a large number of antibiotics (which work only against bacteria but not viruses or fungi) available which can be used topically (like azithromycin, ofloxacin, gentamycin, sulfacetamide and other) and others which can also be taken orally. They are effective (unless the bacteria have developed a resistance to the chosen drug in which case another antibiotic must be used).

Virus infections are caused by viruses. A virus (Latin meaning toxin or poison) is an "organism" that is unable to grow or reproduce outside a host cell. To do this it needs the metabolism of a host cell. Each virus consists of genetic material (either DNA or RNA) within a protective protein coat called a "capsid". It cannot be seen with an ordinary microscope but only with special electron microscopes. Viruses come in different forms and shapes and are classified into different species and strains. Each of them usually infects a special tissue and causes a particular clinical picture. Of these viruses, the herpes and zoster viruses are mostly responsible for eye infections which manifest themselves often as redness, swelling, discomfort/pain and a mucous secretion (usually little or no pus). A viral "pink eye" often disappears after about 10 days without treatment.

Herpes zoster virus which causes chicken pox usually early in life can survive thereafter in the body for many years and may reactivate in adult life causing shingles. The shingles are a painful inflammatory eruption of the skin on the waist, thorax and/or the forehead. The virus also affects the nerves which cause severe pain. Secondarily, the infection can invade the eyes and inflame the cornea which could lead to vision problems. Since viruses invade our cells and use our cellular metabolism, they are more difficult to eradicate. A viral infection must be seen and treated by a health professional who will determine if treatment is indicated or not. There are a number of efficient antiviral drugs available (such as idoxuridine, vidarabine or trifluridine). For shingles, a vaccine is now also available. Many viral infections can be suppressed but often not cured. Viruses have the ability to withdraw into specific human tissues where they are safe from attacks by the immune system. At times of opportunity (stress, illnesses and certain drugs) they emerge from these secure places and attack their preferred tissues again. Individuals suffering from herpes infections know this from their own experiences in that these infections are unfortunately reoccurring.

Fungal infections are caused by fungi which live mostly on plants and human fungal infections are rare and occur mostly in individuals with a compromised immune system (such as in patients suffering from AIDS or being treated with drugs to protect an organ transplant or undergoing chemotherapy for cancer). Fungi are unicellular organisms with their own metabolism. They live from all kinds of organic or even plastic materials (they even grow on plastic contact lenses). They occur in many different forms and shapes, often live in colonies and again are classified into many different species and strains. Some produce antibacterial substances and are a valuable source for the production of many of our antibiotics. Only very few are pathogenic for humans. One fungal infection which can cause serious damage to the eye and even blindness is histoplasmosis. This infection can be contracted from outside cats and dogs. Fungal infections are often difficult to treat but a number of laser procedures and drugs are available (such as amphotericin B, fluconazole, itraconazole or econazole) which often require long term therapy and cause a host of adverse reactions.

Parasitic infections include problems caused by protozoa including amoeba and certain worms. They usually do not present a significant health problem in the USA but are major risk factors in developing countries where they can cause many cases of blindness. Protozoa are unicellular organisms (but they are not bacteria). They live in dirty water which has been in contact with feces. They can also be found in insects (insect bites then transfer these organisms to humans) and animals including cats (which excrete them in their feces and contact with these can also transfer them to us). Again, there are many different species but only a few are dangerous to humans. They withstand the actions of many preservatives and are relatively heat resistant. Swimming in pools, lakes or sea water while wearing contact lenses, storing contact lenses in home made solutions and poor contact lens hygiene can cause a potentially vision threatening infection with a small microbe called acanthamoeba. This problem – acanthamoeba keratitis - is found almost exclusively in contact lens wearers. It manifests itself in severe ocular pain and redness. An advanced acanthamoeba keratitis can cause a white "ring" to cover the iris, as well as redness in the white of the eye. Treatment is difficult and might take one year or longer (drugs used include propamidine, chlorhexidine, miconazole or neomycin) and might sometimes necessitate a corneal transplant. Another problem is toxoplasmosis caused by a protozoan. This microbe is mostly contracted from cats or raw meat. It can also be congenital in that the fetus obtains the parasite from the mother in the womb. The inactive form causes few ocular problems but the active form causes blurred vision, retinal inflammations and eventually retinal scarring. There is no satisfactory treatment although a number of drugs are available (such as atovaquone, azithromycin and bactrim). In addition, steroids are employed to reduce the inflammation.

Worm infections are rare in the USA but are major problems in the developing countries. Some of these worms can affect the eye where they actually live and can be seen. Again, drugs are available but removal of the worms from the eye is most important.

Strabismus. Strabismus, also called squint or heterotropia, is a failure of the eyes to align properly on the object which a person seeks to see. The deviant eye may be directed inward, toward the other eye (cross-eye or esotropia); outward, away from the other eye (walleye, or exotropia); upward (hypertropia); or downward (hypotropia). This misalignment can be transient, usually not observable except during certain times of stress or it can be constant meaning it is always present. This misalignment can be present for all directions or when the gaze is directed in one particular direction. It can be inborn or caused by certain medical conditions or maternal drug abuse during pregnancy. Here, the ocular muscles which move and direct the eyes do not get the proper nerve signals from the brain to function in concert. This problem occurs in about 3 % of children. In some individuals strabismus is self correcting as they grow older but in most it is persistent. As only one eye starts to focus and is used for vision the other eye slowly loses its function and finally ceases to function at all. Thus, strabismus is not just a cosmetic problem but mostly a medical condition where not only double and poor vision are present but also a major vision risk since it can develop into mono-ocular blindness. This medical problem needs attention and consultations with an ophthalmologist, neurologist and optometrist are recommended as early as possible. First several tests have to be performed to determine – if possible - the cause of the problem. The patient will have a thorough eye examination and may be asked to look through a series of prisms to determine the visual differences between the two eyes and the eye muscles will be examined to measure their individual strength. The appropriate treatment for strabismus is dependent on several factors including the patient's age, the cause of the problem, and the type and degree of the eye turn and may include patching, corrective glasses, prisms, or surgery. The better eye can be patched forcing the patient to use and train the weaker eye to see. This seems to be the preferred method at present. The same can be achieved with glasses interfering with the vision of the better eye and favoring the weaker one. In some cases the prognosis is good and the brain will adjust and use the weaker eye properly with vision gradually improving. Drugs can also be used to weaken a specific muscle (like botulinus toxin) or to interfere with vision in the better eye (like atropine). However, many cases eventually will require surgery which is performed under local or general anesthesia. Several different surgical techniques can be used. For instance, an ocular muscle can be weakened or can be strengthened so that the position of the eye will be corrected in order to act in concert with the other eye. In addition, eye exercises to strengthen the weaker eye are often recommended.

Amblyopia. Amblyopia is not strabismus but can occur during this condition. It manifests itself as blurring of vision which can be gradual or sudden in onset and can affect one eye or both eyes. It can be transient or permanent. The disorder may be caused by a brain disorder or by poisoning from several compounds including wood alcohol. One form of amblyopia is known as 'lazy eye" which occurs in about two to three percent of children. Due to incoordination of the eyes the brain receives two pictures which it can not fuse into one and in order to avoid double vision it suppresses the vision of one eye. This can lead to loss of brain function in this area. Treatment of this condition by health professionals is similar to that of strabismus by interfering with vision of the favored eye to train the "lazy" eye to become stronger. If started early prognosis is very good. Treatment includes glasses, patches, drugs and surgery. Also, eye exercises are recommended and can be beneficial in some cases.

Systemic diseases. Various systemic (affecting the body) diseases can also affect the eye. Foremost is perhaps diabetes mellitus or an increase in blood glucose levels either caused by a lack of the glucose lowering hormone insulin or a reduced response of tissues to this hormone. If this problem is not treated or not treated sufficiently, then the high amounts of circulating glucose cause a sprouting of new (unnecessary) blood vessels which can leak blood into the eye and damage the retina. These problems can be prevented or minimized if blood glucose levels in the body are strictly controlled by diet and medications and frequent eye examinations are being performed. Untreated hypertension can affect the optic nerve and cause irreversible damage. This can be prevented if the blood pressure is lowered and controlled. Muscular disorders like Myasthenia gravis can interfere with lid movements and cause drooping eye lids restricting the visual field. Systemic lupus erythematous can cause ulceration of the cornea. Hyperthyroidism can cause bulging eyes. Multiple sclerosis is associated with optic neuritis. Again, treatment of the systemic disease eliminates in many instances such ocular problems.

Drugs given for systemic diseases. A few drugs given for a number of systemic diseases can cause ocular problems which can range from mild to severe. They can prevent the pupil from constricting and cause photophobia or discomfort in bright light (where pupils ordinarily would constrict). In contrast, they can cause pupillary constriction which would interfere with night vision (where the pupils would ordinarily dilate). They could interfere with tear production and cause a dry eye. Some can increase the intraocular pressure or cause cataract formation. Some can cause deposits in the eye or ocular inflammations. Some might cause double vision or problems with moving the eyes properly causing jerky eye movements. In all of these cases the physician must be informed to either change the medication or to prescribe drugs to ease the ocular problems.

Inborn ocular diseases. A number of ocular diseases or disorders are inborn or inherited from our ancestors. They are present in one or both of our parents but the parents can be disease free and be only the carriers of the problem. As we learn more and more about genes we will start to know the genetic cause of such inborn diseases which will then hopefully be followed by discovering the appropriate treatments and cures. At present, we are still in the beginning of this endeavor.

One of these inborn errors is color blindness (although it can also occur due to damage to the retina or brain). The healthy eye has three types of cones – one for green, one for blue and one for red. The other colors are perceived in that more than one of these cones is stimulated. This disorder manifests itself as the inability to distinguish one or more of the three colors red, green, and blue. Color-blind persons may be blind to one, two or all of the colors red, green, and blue and their mixtures. Red-blind persons are ordinarily unable to distinguish between red and green, while blue-blind persons cannot distinguish between blue and yellow. Green-blind persons are unable to see the green part of the spectrum. The cause is that certain types of the cones which are responsible for our color vision are missing or not working at full capacity. Most of these genes which make our cones are located on the x chromosome. A defective x chromosome can but must not cause color blindness. Thus, more men are affected because they have only one x chromosome and if they receive the defective gene they will be color blind. Women have two x chromosomes and if one is defective the other healthy one can take over and prevent color blindness (but these individuals will be silent carrier for the disorder). The women will only be color blind if she inherits two defective x chromosomes. The following scheme shows what happens if a man with sperms carrying either an x or a y chromosome and a women who happens to be a carrier having eggs with either a normal x or defective **x*** will have children (the bold **x*** signifies the defective gene):

If sperm x meets egg x , then the combination will be xx resulting in a normal girl;
If sperm x meets egg **x***, then the combination will be xx* resulting in normal girl who is
       a carrier;
If sperm y meets egg x , then the combination will be yx resulting in a normal boy;
If sperm y meets egg **x***, then the combination will be yx* resulting in a color blind boy.

If the man is color blind (y**x***) and the women is not (xx), then there will be no color blind children but the daughters will be carriers. There are color tests available to determine the exact nature of the disorder. One of them is the Ishihara test where colored dots within other color dots represent a number which can be read by a person with normal color vision but not by a person with color vision defects. There are generally no treatments to cure color deficiencies. However, certain types of tinted filters and contact lenses may help an individual to better distinguish different colors. Optometrists can supply a singular red-tint contact lens to wear in the dominant eye. This may enable the wearer to pass color blindness tests for certain occupations although it may take some time to get used to such lenses. Additionally, computer software has been developed to assist those with visual color difficulties.

Another one of these inborn disorders is retinitis pigmentosa (RP) which is the name for a group of eye diseases. These diseases affect mostly the rods but also the cones which deteriorate and die prematurely. It is passed down from one or both parents. In one type of RP at least fourteen disease-causing genes have already been identified. About 200 000 Americans are currently afflicted. Here, peripheral vision is lost first until the individual can only see a small tunnel of vision straight ahead. Eventual blindness will ensue. The rate of progression and degree of visual loss varies from person to person but most people with RP are legally blind by age forty. Unfortunately, there is no cure available.

Leber's congenital amaurosis or LCA is caused by genetically defective photoreceptor cells which are too light sensitive and are thus prematurely damaged by light. It usually begins affecting sight in early childhood and causes total blindness by the time a patient is thirty. There is no treatment. Recent research has offered some hope. Two teams of researchers used a common cold virus to deliver a normal version of one damaged gene that causes the disease, called RPE65, directly into the eyes of patients. Although both trials were only done to test the safety of the procedure, patients reported they could see a little better afterwards.

Brain. The last and final site of vision – and the most important and complex one – is the brain. As pointed out, there are many areas in the brain which have to work together in harmony to finally produce the complete image or as we see and understand the outside world (which is actually electricity perceived like a picture). If one or more areas are malformed from birth or damaged through an accident (trauma, penetrating wounds), a stroke, poisoning (carbon monoxide) or alcoholism, then specific visual deficits occur. These deficits are often mild and only slightly disturbing but can also be very severe, bizarre and greatly interfering with life. These problems are often not easily understood by most individuals.

A condition which occurs in a relatively large number of individuals at different degrees is dyslexia. Dyslexia is an inability or pronounced difficulty to read or spell in spite of otherwise normal intellectual functions. It is a chronic neurological disorder and primary symptoms include seeing letters and words in reversed sequences and reversals of words and letters in the person's speech. There are many different forms of this disorder. A mild and usually reversible type is that some children see letters or numbers reversed like a ⌐ as a Γ or as a ⌐. The brain has yet to learn to make the proper adjustments of the received inverted images and it will usually do so in due time. In some cases, the problem is more severe involving entire words and will not correct itself over time. Reading and spelling exercises will help some and make this problem more manageable. Another problem more severe is "letter or word blindness" or alexia. In the case of total alexia, an individual will recognize numbers and geometrical patters easily but not letters and cannot read words. Partial word blindness permits the individual to recognize letters but only to read concrete nouns like "inn" or "tool" but not abstract words like "in" or "too". This results from damage to a specific brain area often caused by a stroke.

Damage to the primary visual cortex can cause a blind spot or scotoma. Individuals will not see a part of the visual field. Some individuals will fill in this blind spot involuntarily. For instance, if they look at a picture on the wall with their blind spot they will not see the picture but might see the color of the wallpaper – here, the brain "assumes" it must be wallpaper since nothing is seen and it then fills in color and pattern of the wall paper.

Malfunction of other brain areas (the left occipital and temporal lobes) causes a condition referred to as visual agnosia which includes the inability to identify, draw or copy common objects including sub-divisions where faces can not be recognized or remembered. For instance, a copy of an anchor would result in a cross consisting of crooked lines.

A genetic disorder is William's syndrome. Here, individuals cannot draw from memory or assemble pictures correctly. When asked to draw a dog they might draw the body parts but place them in the wrong places.

In the case of the loss of face recognition, patients will see the face of the spouse but do not recognize it as the face of the spouse or they will look into a mirror but do not recognize their own face and see a stranger each time they look into a mirror. The inability to recognize faces is called "face blindness" or prosopagnosia.Other disorders are where patients cannot identify objects or cannot recognize a whole image although they recognize clearly individual details of it. These patients still have the functional areas which "see" objects but have lost the functions of areas which provide meaning and recognition to the visual images and, therefore, are not able to make a meaningful association. This is mostly confined to the visual senses while otherwise they have intact recognition of what they hear or feel   However, these recognition defects can also occur with sounds or touch where, for instance, patients will hear a voice but can not recognize the person who speaks although it is a familiar voice.

If damage occurs in another brain area, they will be blind but actually can "see" but are not aware that they can see. For instance, such a blind patient might be shown a pencil and asked what they see. They will respond that they do not see anything. But when asked to grasp it, they will reach for the pencil and grasp it properly. They will walk down a maze without bumping into obstacles. This condition has been named "blind sight".

If damage occurs still in another area, these individuals have trouble judging motion since this might occur not in the usual smooth way but in a strobe-like or abrupt fashion. This is sometimes called "motion blindness". They are afraid to cross a road without a stop light since they cannot judge correctly the speed of oncoming cars. They will see the car in the distance and then the car all of a sudden in front of them. They will pour water into a cup but the flow of water appears like a solid column of water.

Sometimes blind people will make up for lost visual impressions. Such a patient might sometimes "see" the dark field filled with hallucinations – sometimes cartoons and sometimes people and animals. This is referred to as the "Charles Bonnet Syndrome". It is like the brain wants to "see" something and if it does not receive real input from the world it just makes up its own visual images. This occurs sometimes in people who lost their vision due to glaucoma, AMD or retinal diabetes.

Damage to another area causes the 'neglect syndrome". These patients see perfectly well but just show a complete indifference or neglect of one side of their visual field. For instance, they will neglect the left side and groom the right side of the body or will eat the food from the right side but not from the left side of the plate. However, when forced they can notice objects on their left side.

Damage yet to another area will cause the "Capras Delusion". Here, these individuals will see, for instance, their parents but will not recognize them as parents but will think of them as imposters. They will say they look like my parents but actually are not my parents.

In the "Frigoli Confusion", patients with damage to another specific area will see the same face everywhere. For instance, this patient will see the face of every man as the face of his or her father.

Patients suffering from dorsal simultanagnosia, again caused by a stroke or trauma to the head, have restriction of view. They have a full visual field of their eyes but the brain can only "see" one object or a part of one object at a time which will sometimes suddenly slip from their sight.

Yet damage to another area can give rise to acchromatopsia or a loss to see colors in the brain (although the cones in the retina are normal and healthy). These individuals will see the world gray and cannot even imagine colors how they actually are.

There are individuals who have lost a limb. If, for instance, one hand is lost it cannot be seen anymore but it can still be felt by them (because the area in the brain which is responsible for this hand is still functioning and might not "know" that it is missing). This is referred to as 'phantom sensation" and sometimes the missing hand can hurt very much which is then called "phantom pain". Such a patient can sometimes developed a "picture" of the missing hand on the upper left arm and when this part would be touched he would feel as if his left hand would be touched. Unfortunately, little can be done to help these patients at this time if they experience "phantom pain" although a variety of behavioral methods are available which can bring some relief in milder cases.

Sometimes a mental problem or disorder can cause visual problems. Hysterical blindness, now called Conversion Blindness, is a loss of vision which can occur after extreme stress. A person, for instance, can lose vision if he or she sees a terrible event like one's child being killed in a car accident. This type of blindness can resolve by itself or psychotherapy can be successfully employed. People suffering from schizophrenia might have visual hallucinations (although auditory hallucinations are more common) and might be seeing and talking, for instance, to people who do not exist. Antipsychotic drugs are now available which can be helpful to correct this problem (as well as other psychotic problems) in a large number of these patients. A person with anorexia nervosa has a deep fear of gaining weight. This person thinks a lot about food but restricts food intake drastically and becomes soon severely underweight. One of the causes is a distorted self image in that the person sees and perceives herself (most patients are female) as fat when actually she is very thin. It is common that such persons may see another person and think "I wish I could be as skinny as them" while in reality they are actually much skinnier. Although some treatments are available including medications and psychotherapy, they are only helpful in some individuals.

The brain can play even more surprising and weirder tricks on vision like in the case of a person with multiple personalities or Dissociative Identity Disorder. In this case a single person displays two or more distinct and independent identities or personalities each taking at certain times control of the individual's behavior and displaying his or her own pattern of perceiving and interacting with the environment. Recently, such a person was reported where one or more of these personalities were "blind". During these "blind" phases, the individual could not see and physiological tests revealed that there was indeed no activity to be found in the visual brain areas. Such a condition is very difficult to treat and psychological therapies are mostly unsuccessful.

A visual peculiarity is synesthesia – it is estimated to occur in about 1 in 500 000 individuals -which is not a disabling but actually an appreciated phenomenon by most of these individuals. This condition refers to the perception of a concomitant sensation other than the one being stimulated. For instance, these individuals can hear colors or can see sounds. One such individual remarked: I see a 3 as the black font it is typed in, but in my mind I also see it as completely yellow, and S is green in my mind, while O is white. Famous composers like Franz Liszt and Nikolai Rimsky-Korsakov saw specific colors when they heard certain notes or cords- it has been claimed that they argued bitterly with each other about which color belonged to which cord. This condition can be inborn (about 1 in 23 persons) or caused by unknown circumstances. Certain psychedelic compounds like LSD or mescaline can also cause this condition. The most likely cause is that nerve pathways for individual sensations which usually run separate to the brain do cross-stimulate each other. Sounds travel along the auditory pathway can in these cases also stimulate the visual pathway so that sounds are heard and colors are seen (because the visual centers in the brain respond to electrical signals regardless if they originated in the eye or were initiated at a different place).

If a person suffers from extreme epilepsy which does not respond to medications, surgery is sometimes employed. The cause of epilepsy is the dangerous spread of localized, normal electrical activity to other parts of or the entire brain. In order to prevent the spread from one hemisphere to the other one, the connection between both brain hemispheres is sometimes severed. Such an individual when shown an image in his or her left visual field (that is, the left half of what both eyes see) projecting to the right side of the rbain will be unable to name what he or she has seen. This is because the speech-control center in most people is in the left side of the brain and the visual image from the left visual field can not be sent to the right side of the brain. Those with the speech control center in the right side will experience similar symptoms when an image is presented in the right visual field. The person can, however, pick up and show recognition of an object (one within the left overall visual field) with their right hand, since that hand is controlled by the left side of the brain.

Medications to treat ocular problems. In many cases, physicians and optometrists prescribe medications to treat certain of these ocular problems. Unfortunately, many patients are worried to use medications as recommended because they are afraid of adverse reactions. While drugs are now well tested and very effective, they nevertheless carry a certain risk which in most cases is relatively small but in some instances can be unfortunately serious and even life threatening. Thus, why should these drugs then be used if they can be dangerous? The choice of a drug is based on the

BENEFIT outweighing the RISK

principle. The physician, ophthalmologist or optometrist determines your benefit versus your risk in using a particular drug. For instance, an eye disease if untreated may lead in fifty % of all cases to vision impairment or even complete vision loss. A drug which might cure this disease, however, carries a risk of five % to cause another serious visual problem. Thus, the health professional weighs the benefits versus risks and decides – as most of us would agree – to use the drug ssince it will prevent forty-five percent of the original visual problems. Do you ever consider when you drive your car to go shopping or to a movie that about 40 000 healthy individuals are killed and 100 000 are seriously injured in car accidents each year? Apparently, we accept this risk since we like to go shopping or to the movies hoping nothing will happen to us. Accept this also when using a drug – I will be careful and I will not experience serious adverse reactions. But also watch out for adverse reactions if they occur because many of them when recognized early can be reversed just by stopping the drug and switching to another one. On the other hand, patients sometimes ask for drugs and are disappointed if the physician does not prescribe a drug. The physician must have determined that the benefits in this case do not outweigh the risks and that the use of an antibiotic, for instance, would not be helpful, could cause an adverse reaction and will only increase the chance of creating another drug resistant bacterial strain.

To optimize the beneficial effects and to minimize the adverse reactions, it is important to follow drug instructions as closely as possible. Some drugs supposed to be taken two hours before a meal can loose their effectiveness if taken with a meal. A drug which is supposed to be taken with a meal and is consumed on an empty stomach can cause severe stomach problems. Follow the instructions closely and the risk of adverse reactions will be reduced. Do not smoke when taking a contraceptive medication – if the individual nevertheless smokes her chances of experiencing a stroke increases manifold. Adverse reactions might not be caused by a drug but by the patient per se. A peculiarity in the biological make-up of the individual which will be of no importance in every day life and the individual might not even be aware of it if no drug is used, can be a cause of health problems if a drug is taken. Most individuals enjoy peanuts which are healthy and taste good (except adding weight if too many of them are consumed). However, a few individuals might experience an allergic reaction or in a very few instances even death. This is not the fault of the peanuts but due to a special immunological peculiarity of this person. This also holds true for drugs – while penicillins are well tolerated by most individuals a few will show allergic reactions and the drug must be stopped.

In contrast to a few decades ago, drugs to-day are well researched, precisely manufactured and extensive experience is available on their beneficial and detrimental effects. The Food and Drug Administration only allows drugs to enter the market if the company can provide extensive data as to their benefits and risks – which can cost the company 500 million dollars and more over a period of about 10 years before they can market the drug and make money. Later, beneficial and detrimental effects are monitored as well and the Food and Drug Administration can remove a drug if it shows not the expected benefits or exhibits to many unacceptable side effects – and the agency has done so in the past and will do so in the future. Today, drugs are safer than driving a car. Ask yourself or your friends if they know somebody who has died in a car accident and then ask the same question about a person who has died definitively of a drug induced death (excluding of course suspicions, intuitions or feelings of such occurrences).

But be aware of alternative medications unless recommended by a physician or optometrist. Many of these herbal preparations, minerals and vitamins do not deliver what they promise - often using reckless and shady advertisements and unsafe manufacturing procedures. Some of them can actually be harmful. In contrast to prescription and over-the-counter drugs, they are not under the control of the Food and Drug Administration (except they must state the content) and do not have to prove that they are effective and safe – and most are not effective as shown in later trials. Some can adversely interact with prescription drugs and their use must be mentioned to a physician before he or she prescribes a drug. These products carry a warning label which says that this product is **not** to be used to diagnose, prevent, treat or cure any disease! Thus, the manufacturer actually states that this product is ineffective as a medication – why do people then buy it????

Another albeit much rarer problem is faith. There are still some people who refuse medical treatment and choose prayers and faith instead. Jehovah's witnesses refuse blood transfusions because the Bible says that blood can not be digested and this includes its storage and transfusion. Although it is rare but instances surf once in a while that parents refuse treatment for their children out of religious beliefs with the unfortunate outcome of their deaths. These parents can be charged with reckless endangerment of their children's death. The court faces difficult decisions with these religious and ethical problems and apparently no satisfactory laws have been developed to cover these cases as of yet.

Today's drugs are powerful but must be handled with care. They and surgery (only made possible with the help of anesthetic drugs) have markedly increased the quality of life and our longevity and have prevented or restored vision impairment and loss in countless individuals.

How to Take Care of Our Eyes

Our eyes and our vision are one of the most important functions of our body which let us enjoy life to the fullest. Thus, we must take care of them and not squander our eyesight away. Here are a few suggestions how to take care of our eyesight well into old age. These suggestions are based on recommendations made by professional societies representing ophthalmologists, optometrists and opticians as well as by the National Institutes of Health, the Mayo Clinic and similar reputable sources.

In general, it can be said what is good for the body is good for the eyes. Good eyes in a healthy body are the ultimate goal while good eyes in a sick body or bad eyes in a healthy body are poor alternatives. Thus, the golden rule to preserve good health and reduce health problems for the body and eyes to a minimum is: eat a well balanced diet, exercise regularly, have an optimistic outlook on life, seek periodic medical check-ups and eye examinations and adhere strictly to prescribed or recommended medical treatments.

The diet we consume is important because this is what keeps us alive and provides the energy to fulfill our daily activities. It is well known that improper diets or one sided diets can lead to a number of diseases caused by a lack of necessary nutrients, vitamins or minerals. A diet deficient in vitamin A can lead to difficulties seeing in dim light. All this can be prevented if we are fortunate enough to have the opportunity to eat right (which unfortunately does not exist in all parts of the world) and which sadly is not followed by a large number of people. In addition, studies have shown over and over again that a good diet used in moderation to maintain normal body weight will provide for a healthy body including healthy eyes and a longer life. Such a body is also able to correct some internal problems which might arise during our life time as well as external problems such as fighting infections more effectively. What is now the appropriate diet? This depends on the individual and might vary from individual to individual. Individuals prone to have high blood pressure, high cholesterol or glucose levels which affect adversely the blood vessels in the body and in the eyes should reduce their intake of salt, cholesterol and/or sugar/carbohydrate containing foods. These precautions are not that important with individuals with low blood pressure, low cholesterol and low glucose levels. Furthermore, the advice offered by nutritionists varies as more and more research is being done. Thus, a mixture of low fat meats including fish, unsaturated fats and oils and carbohydrates with a number of healthy servings of vegetables and fruits are recommended. Here, dark vegetables and fruits and fish including omega-3 fish oil supplementation seem to be the favorites. One or two glasses of wine or a cocktail also have been claimed to be beneficial.

Recently, supplementation of the diet with vitamins and minerals to prevent diseases or even to cure diseases of the body and the eyes has received a lot of publicity. Can these supplements indeed help our eyes and prevent ocular problems? There is little evidence that this is so for the average healthy eye and many previous recommendations to take large doses of certain vitamins and minerals in addition to a balanced diet have been rescinded in the mean time. Multivitamins once thought to be quite beneficial have been found not to provide the benefits once thought although taking a tablet 2- 3 times a week might not help but it certainly cannot hurt. Most nutritionists feel that our vitamins and minerals should come from the diet. At present there is no evidence that vitamin or mineral supplementations – contrary to the claims of many manufacturers and rumors – will prevent the occurrence of eye problems. Thus, for individuals with healthy eyes a good balanced diet with lots of vegetables and fruits are sufficient (safe your money!). To those who still believe in the benefits of large doses of vitamins and minerals a word of caution is in order – while small amounts of both are absolutely necessary for life and any lack of either of them can lead to deficiency diseases, large amounts of some (e.g. vitamin A and D, beta carotene, iron) can be dangerous and toxic to the body. Thus, caution is advised. This, of course, as outlined above for healthy eyes is different if there are health problems and certain minerals and vitamins taken in larger doses do indeed help somewhat individuals with ocular problems, for instance, for reducing the progression of macular degeneration (but these vitamins and minerals will not prevent the onset of this problem).

In addition, a lot of attention has been lately placed on alternative medications such as herbal preparations. Some of the problems with these preparations have been outlined before but are highlighted here again because people do waste a lot of money on them and might often do more harm than good. The big question is: how effective are these "medications". Most of these "medications" have never been tested for efficacy (do they indeed work as promised in scientific and clinical trials and do they provide a definite health benefit) and, worse, for safety (are they safe because the claim that they come from nature is not sufficient since nature contains a fair number of poisonous plants). They rely on catch phrases in large print like: *no chemicals but all natural products* (natural products are chemicals); *have been used by Chinese people for ages* (so why is the life expectancy in China so much lower than in our country?); *they help the immune system or other problems* (they do not say: they have been shown to strengthen the immune system or cure the common cold – only "help" which could range from insignificant to significant). Important is the statement which is on all bottles but not read by most buyers and users because it is in extra fine print: "*This product is not intended to diagnose, treat, cure or prevent any disease.* The manufacturer clearly states herewith that this product is ineffective – and yet people buy these products at the tune of billions of dollars every year. If a car is advertised as: this vehicle is not intended to be driven on a highway or street – who would buy the car? In addition, surveys of these products by the government have revealed that most indeed contain what is written on the box but that they vary often markedly in strength that is some contain very little of the active ingredients while others contain more – thus, one never knows how much one gets. Cases have also been cited where unscrupulous manufacturers adulterated their products often with toxic materials.

They get away easily with these tactics because Congress legislated that the FDA must strictly control prescription drugs as to efficacy and toxicity as well as content and dosage while these herbal preparations are only controlled as to content (as long as there is a bit of a supposedly beneficial component in a preparation, it fulfills the letters of the law). Furthermore, their manufacturing processes are poorly supervised and controlled. Unfortunately, a fair number of serious poisonings and deaths have been reported from the use of some of these substances. The last warning: they can seriously interfere with the action of some prescription drugs and can render some less effective and others more dangerous. Thus, physicians must be informed if such herbal products are being taken.

Vitamins, minerals and alternative medications should not be used without proper advice. If you use the computer to search for vitamin, mineral or alternative medications, go for web sites which end in ".edu" (university related) or ".gov" (government agencies or National Institutes of Health related). These web sites you can trust while others might be correct or not in their recommendations but often just want to sell products and make money.

Also, homeopathic products are now making their way back into the market including products supposedly helpful for the eye. A homeopathic product is the invention of a late medieval physician by the name of Hahnemann who lived about 1800. This physician hypothesized that diluting a solution of a natural substance until almost nothing or indeed nothing is left, would increase its strength and could heal diseases. This is "magic" and scientific studies have not shown this to be true. It is like taking a shot of whiskey and diluting it 10 times in a row so that almost no whiskey is left and when consumed would make you more drunk than the original whiskey. The opinion of this author based on a surveillance of these preparations for decades is: stay away until the manufacturers are forced to study their products scientifically and clinically and can provide definite proof of their efficacy and relative safety.

The next proven factor in staying in good health and living longer is exercise. The benefits of exercise have been well documented and cannot be ignored. Exercise can be performed by all age groups albeit at different levels of intensity. You are never too young or too old to exercise. Just to mention a few benefits: it lowers blood pressure and cholesterol levels which benefit the blood vessels in the body and the eyes. It reduces stress, keeps the weight down, improves sleep, delivers more oxygen to body tissues and improves mood. Exercise can, for instance, start with 30 min of walking briskly, mowing the lawn, dancing, swimming or bicycling 3-4 times a week. If walking is boring, listening to music or to books on tape can be very helpful to pass the time. In the latter case, you can now choose from a wide variety of CDs ranging from crime stories to educational material. Stretching and weight training can strengthen your body and improve your fitness level. Take the stairs instead of the elevator, go for a walk during your coffee break or lunch or walk quickly part of the way to or from work. If more strenuous exercise is intended like in a fitness center or on home based equipment, consult with a health professional before to find out what you can do and what you should not do. Many injuries are reported each year where people did the wrong exercises or did the right exercises wrongly. But start and/or continue to exercise the benefits are well documented. It improves the health of our blood vessels in the body and those in the eyes and brain.

Scientific studies have strongly suggested that emotionally well balanced people with an optimistic outlook on life are in better health and recover better from surgery or diseases. Evidence is available that people who are depressed, anxious or stressed are more prone to diseases, infections and other health problems. Studies in animals and humans have demonstrated that stress can significantly weaken the immune system and predispose to infections as well as cancer. In addition, such a person may not feel like exercising, eating nutritious foods or taking drugs as described and to make matters worse might resort to the use of excessive amounts of alcohol, smoke more or abuse illegal drugs. An optimistic outlook in life maintains and improves body health including the health of our eyes and brains.

Most people are born fortunately with healthy eyes or only with some minor problems like short sightedness which can be easily corrected. It is now important to keep these eyes healthy, preserve vision and protect them from being damaged or injured. Below are a few suggestions to preserve our healthy eyesight as long as possible.

First and utmost, it is strongly recommended that individuals have their eyes checked by an optometrist or ophthalmologist, in particular as they grow older. It has been estimated that about 20% of Americans do not have regular eye check-ups. Some of them might be harboring silent "killers" which will affect their vision later on and which in many cases could have been easily prevented. If individuals have eye glasses then this will be done each time the refraction of the glasses is being checked. If no glasses are worn then individuals should make their own appointments. There are problems which can slowly damage the eyes and reduce eyesight which individuals are not aware of until it is too late. Glaucoma is one case in point. The pressure in the eyes of such individuals increases slowly without being noticed (similar to high blood pressure which is also not felt). There are no signs or symptoms to warn the person that there is a problem. Perhaps later peripheral vision becomes impaired but most people compensate for this loss by turning their heads more frequently. Finally, vision becomes more and more constricted and an ophthalmologist will then be consulted. Unfortunately, this physician can only diagnose the problem and can prevent further damage but cannot undo the damage already done. A visit much earlier for a regular check-up would have nipped the problem in the bud and vision would have remained unchanged. Similarly, if floaters in the eye are noted – they manifest themselves like little insects flying in front of your eyes – and if flashes of light occur for no apparent reason, a quick visit to the ophthalmologist is indicated because this could signal a retinal detachment. In most cases, this problem can be solved promptly without ocular damage but if untreated for a few days serious vision problems can ensue. Thus, even if vision seems good and no eye problems are present or noticeable, check-ups are highly recommended to preserve good vision in particular if there is a family history of eye diseases. According to the American Academy of Ophthalmology, children with a family history of childhood vision problems should be screened for common childhood eye problems before the age of 5. Adults between the ages of 40 to 65 should have an eye exam every two to four years. Adults over the age of 65 should have an eye exam at least every one to two years.

But there are a number of other precautions which all of us should heed and pay attention to. Most are simple and constitute minor inconveniences but the payout in terms of eye protection and preservation can be tremendous.

Sometimes a foreign body like a small grain of sand or dirt can enter the eye during our daily activities. There is little what can be done to prevent such happenings. Furthermore, certain ways to remove it can be dangerous. Symptoms include a feeling that there is "something" in the eye, the eyes become watery and red and a scratchy feeling occurs when blinking. This should not be ignored since a foreign body in the eye can scratch the surface of the cornea. If a small foreign body adheres to the outside of the eye and did not penetrate the eye, do not try to remove it physically except by washing and flushing. Tweezers or other instruments can scratch the surface of the eye, especially the cornea. If it is lodged under the contact lens then the lens should be removed quickly before it can scratch the cornea. Gently pour a steady stream of lukewarm water (do not heat the water) from a pitcher or faucet over the eye. Flush for up to 15 minutes, checking the eye every 5 minutes to see if the foreign body has been flushed out. Washing the eye will usually remove the foreign object. If no relief is obtained an ophthalmologist or optometrist should be consulted.

Many eye injuries which occur during work or during sports activities could have been easily prevented. It is estimated that each day 2,000 workers in this country alone suffer eye injuries on the job. Many tools and machineries contribute to these eye injuries if used improperly and/or without safety glasses. Hand and power tools such as saws, drills and sanders present a danger to eyes when precautions are not taken. However, eye injuries occur not only at work but in the house as well when using caustic chemicals or various tools or when mowing the lawn. Many of these injuries could have been prevented if the right type of protective eyewear like goggles had been used. It is estimated that 90 percent of all eye injuries could have been prevented or minimized through the use of proper protective eyewear. Thus, it is imperative – even for quick and small jobs at work or at home - to wear protective goggles which can be easily obtained in any hardware store. While it might sometimes present itself as a minor inconvenience it will definitively prevent major inconvenience and eye damage in the future.

Similarly, eye injuries can occur while engaging in many sports. It has been estimated that up to 40 000 minor to serious sport related eye injuries occur each year. A baseball, racquetball or tennis ball hitting the unprotected eye can cause significant damage. Use of goggles with polycarbonate lenses which do not splinter at impact could have prevented most of these injuries.

If such injuries occur, ophthalmologists make the following recommendations. If a minor blow to the eye occurs, a cold compress should be applied without putting pressure on the eye. Crushed ice in a plastic bag can be taped to the forehead to rest gently on the injured eye. In more severe cases or if significant pain, reduced vision or discoloration of the eye is present, medical help is needed quickly since any of these symptoms could mean internal eye damage. Penetrating trauma where the eye is pierced by a sharp or pointed object such as a knife, pair of scissors or any other sharp and pointed object is much more serious. A large object such as a knife or a pair of scissors must be taken out but a smaller object should not be removed. Also, a contact lens should not be removed. The eye can be bandaged loosely without pressure on the eye on the way to see an ophthalmologist as soon as possible. This is an emergency. The ophthalmologist will then take the proper steps in removing the object and provide the individual with medications to prevent an inflammation and infection. One of the most serious injuries of the eye is a chemical burn. Damage caused could be minor and temporary such as by hairspray or it can be severe and possibly blinding caused, for instance, by alkalis and acids. When a chemical injury occurs, the eyes should be flooded immediately for at least ten minutes with any neutral fluid available such as water or soda pop to minimize the damage. After irrigation, emergency medical care should be sought at once.

Frequent hits to the head – like during boxing – can lead to a retinal detachment. But even frequent minor bumps – like during headers in soccer or collusions in football – can eventually hasten a retinal detachment in susceptible individuals. If there is a family history of such a problem, frequent visits to a health professional or choosing a different sport is recommended.

It is also strongly recommended that eyes should be shielded from bright sun light.

Harmful ultraviolet light has been shown to speed up the development of cataracts and macular degeneration and it can cause abnormal thickening or growths to form on the eye. Melanoma can also occur in the eye. At risk are people who spend long hours in the sun, who had cataract surgery or who are taking certain medications such as tranquilizers, tetracycline and diuretics. Furthermore, smoking increases your risk of getting cataracts and macular degeneration. Smoke is also a major irritant to people with the dry eye syndrome.

Many infections in the eye like a blepharitis or conjunctivitis are transmitted from the hand to the eyes. If a person is prone to such infections, the best prevention is to wash hands frequently with soap (do not use soap with antibiotics – they are not as effective as thought and its use can lead to the emergence of resistant bacteria). Washing the hands should last at least thirty seconds. Also avoid touching the eyes unnecessarily which reduces the risk of eye infections.

While many individuals use contact lenses without problems, these devices can carry some risks. Following guidelines, instructions and the advice of the health professional strictly can prevent many eye problems from occurring. Since there are different types of contact lenses there are different instructions as to their uses. Sometimes contact lenses are worn too long or are cleaned with the wrong solutions. Never, never put the contact lens into your mouth when repositioning a lens which had slipped. This is a major source of eye infections. One major problem is when the lens slips off the eye. In most cases, it can be repositioned. But it sometimes goes under the eyelid and cannot be repositioned on the cornea. Here, the individual might have to seek professional help (it will do no harm if it is under the eyelid for a number of hours). A particular nasty problem is a small single celled microorganism called acanthamoeba as mentioned before. Washing lenses and lens cases with tap water or homemade saline made from well water and swimming with lenses in contaminated waters allow these microorganisms to adhere to contact lenses. They are then transferred from the lenses to the eye and even the tiniest scratch or abrasion on the surface of the cornea allows the amoeba to get inside the eye, where they multiply and start to destroy ocular tissue. Adhering to strict recommendations how to use and clean contact lenses avoids easily these and other problems.

Pets are nice to have but they can be a source of significant danger if not properly checked by a veterinarian. Toxoplasmosis caused by a single-celled parasite called Toxoplasma gondii is usually acquired by contact with cats and their feces or with raw or undercooked meat. The U.S. Centers for Disease Control and Prevention (CDC) estimates that more than 60 million people in the United States may carry this parasite, but very few have symptoms because a healthy immune system usually keeps them under control. The babies of women who were exposed to the parasites within a few months of pregnancy are at an increased risk. According to the U.S. National Institutes of Health, pregnant women who contract the parasite have a 40% chance of transmitting it to their unborn child. Most infants have no symptoms at birth, but a certain percentage may be born with or develop shortly after birth significant eye or brain damage. Again, a visit with the pets to the veterinarian, washing hands frequently and cooking meat well can easily prevent these problems.

Parents of school-age children should be alert for signs of abnormal visual development or coordination problems. According to eye professionals, it is important to observe young children and recognize abnormal ocular signs and symptoms. They include frequent inward, outward, upward, or downward turning of an eye, excessive tearing of the eyes, excessive blinking, obvious favoring of one eye, squinting or frequent closing of one eye, covering of one eye with hands when looking at objects, drifting of one eye when looking at objects, swollen or crusted eyelids, unusual redness of the eyes or eyelids, bumps, sores or styes on or around the eyelids, unusual position of the eyelids or drooping eyelids, excessive rubbing or touching of the eyes, avoidance of bright lights, frequent complaints of eye strain, turning or tilting of the head when looking at objects, tendency to bump into objects on one side, frequent headaches, fatigue, nausea, or dizziness, below expected eye-hand coordination, losing place while reading, holding reading materials unusually close, making frequent reversals when reading or writing, using fingers to maintain position while reading, omitting or confusing easy words when reading and/or performing below average in any activities. If one or more of these symptoms and signs occur in a child, then a visit to an eye professional is strongly advised.

Also be aware that many systemic diseases (affecting the body) not only affect various organs in the body but can have adverse effects on the eyes as well. Many of such diseases if recognized early or regularly checked and treated effectively can markedly delay the onset of bodily harm and severe ocular problems. For instance, medical conditions like hypertension and diabetes mellitus are thought by many to only affect the body can also give rise to severe ocular problems and the eyes of such patients must be checked regularly by the physician or an ophthalmologist or optometrist. Both conditions if untreated or only poorly controlled can lead to the sprouting of unwanted blood vessels in the eyes which start to leak blood and damage nerve fibers. Vision will become impaired and even blindness can ensue. There are other systemic diseases which can also adversely affect the eyes. One problem is that many of them do not present themselves with warning signals but do their damage silently and health problems are only noticed when it is often too late. Thus, regular visits to a physician are indicated to recognize and treat such problems as soon as possible.

If ocular problems are experienced by an individual who has regular eye examinations, then this individual must often use his or her own judgment in what to do. It might not be necessary to visit a health professional at the first sign of a minor eye irritation (but it must be remembered that sudden vision loss, a "curtain" or "shade" appearing before one eye or light flashes are emergency signs which dictate a trip to an ophthalmologist or emergency room as soon as possible). The best advice is to leave the eye untreated if problems arise. Do not use over-the-counter drugs on your own since this can mask a serious problem and can delay proper treatment. If no improvement is experienced during the next days or the eyes get worse, see a health professional as soon as possible. This visit might reveal a minor problem which needs no treatment. Do not be disappointed if the ophthalmologist or optometrist (depending on the state optometrists can now treat certain eye diseases) does not prescribe a drug but tells you just to use warm or cold compresses or wash your eye with an eye friendly, usually a baby, shampoo or soap. In these cases, drugs have been found not to help. Use of an unnecessary antibiotic is now being blamed as one of the sources of the development of drug resistant bacteria. However, such a visit might reveal a major problem. If a medication is prescribed use the medication as indicated.

If a prescription drug has been prescribed use it exactly as outlined in the package insert or as advised by the ophthalmologist. Proper use enhances the beneficial effects and reduces often adverse reactions. The reason is very simple. If, for instance, a drug is applied, to the eye, it will reach a certain effective concentration on the outside or inside of the eye and then leaves the eye again. At this time, it is necessary to apply the next dose so that the concentration of the drug on or in the eye always remains effective. If the drug is applied too frequently the concentration will rise above the desired concentration and might be harmful. If the drug is applied at too long an interval then the effective concentration will sink below its effective level and, for instance, the bacteria can grow again. If a drug should be applied to the eye, for instance, 4 times a day, the best way is to make a schedule: I get up at 7:00 am and apply the first dose. The next dose should be applied at noon and the next at 5:00 pm. The last dose should be applied at 10.00 pm before going to bed. Thus, write these times on a piece of paper and place it on a visible place. A schedule like this will remind you of a particular time since you might have forgotten when the last dose was applied. If you forgot to use an application then the rule of thumb is as follows: if you remember shortly after the missed time then use the missed application. If you remember shortly before the next dose then skip the missed application.

In conclusion, a few words of hope and warning. Unfortunately, some individuals are born with severe eye problems or blind for whom no help exists today. However, individuals born with certain eye problems or predispositions to develop such problems during their life time can now be successfully either cured or their healthy vision can be prolonged considerably. Individuals with healthy eyes are still at risk in that they might damage their eyes without their control like in unforeseen accidents or infections but more often due to neglect and ignorance. It is imperative to have eye examinations in particular as one ages. As outlined, many eye problems progress without warning signs. Furthermore, many healthy eyes get damaged and even lost because they were not properly shielded. Protective eyewear or goggles must not only be worn as mandated by law during certain manufacturing procedures but also at home when using household chemicals, tools or the lawn mower or during certain sport activities. It is easy to preserve our vision as long as possible by following a healthy life style, having frequent eye examinations and follow strictly therapy instructions if indicated.

History of Vision and the Healthy and Diseased Eye

Introduction. Today, we know a great deal about the origin of light and the structures of the eye and the brain and have obtained a relative good idea how our vision works or how we see the world around us. We also can now diagnose, understand and treat a large number of ocular diseases and can preserve or restore vision in many individuals with ocular problems. However, this knowledge did not arrive over night but is based on the work, research, speculations and theories of the past. The great scholar Isaac Newton wrote (paraphrasing an older quote): *"If I have seen further, it is by standing on the shoulders of giants"* stressing the importance of previous research and scientific efforts which made his own work and discoveries possible.

Thus, the following will - for the historically inclined reader - provide a few glimpses into the past and show how this scientific and medical knowledge about light, the eye and brain and vision in health and disease slowly at first but explosively later on developed over the centuries. We might laugh at some of the earlier vision theories and medical treatment modalities but we must recognize that previous scholars and physicians had only their eyes available as scientific tools since scientific instruments like the microscope and other more highly developed scientific devices were not available at first and were only invented later on. Furthermore, religious considerations, social and political situations and ancient traditions and beliefs sometimes interfered or conflicted with the study and progress of science and medicine. Nevertheless, these early observations and theories provided the stepping stones for our knowledge of today which again is a stepping stone for further knowledge to come in the future.

History provides a colorful picture of the leaps and bounds of the progression of scientific and medical knowledge which was also interspersed with regressions into blind alleys. It shows how prejudice often did hamper progress and how courageous scientists and physicians had to struggle against ignorance and false beliefs – sometimes at their own personal risks – to advance scientific and medical knowledge.

The history of our healthy and diseased eyes and how we see encompasses basically four major scientific and medical areas – light and its very nature, the basic anatomical structures of the eye and the brain, the visual process per se and the nature of ocular diseases and their treatments. All of them are, of course, intricately interwoven and depending on each other.

Light. In the beginning of time – about 14 billion years ago – the universe was dark. Darkness was everywhere. At about 4 to 5 billion years ago the sun and earth started to come into existence. The sun became the first source of light by sending some mysterious waves to earth. Only after the advent of organisms with eyes and brains around 500 million years ago, which could convert these mysterious waves into "light", did light appear for the first time and these creatures could now see their surroundings. Thus, these waves radiating from the sun were crucial for us and animals to develop (as mentioned in the chapter of: How animals do see) and to see our surroundings.

About 400,000 BCE another 'light" source – that is another source of these mysterious waves - appeared on our earth when Homo erectus discovered fire most likely by accident such as a fire being set by lightening. All matter hotter than about 700 degrees sends out such waves which can be converted by eyes and brains into light and is said to be incandescent. Early humans must have cultivated the fire until they started to make it themselves like rubbing two wood sticks together or by hitting iron containing stones against each other. Soon torches, lamps burning animal or vegetable fats and oils were invented and used. This was the source of "light" during the night for many centuries to come. The fire which would light the night was of course also used to warm us when the climate was cold or winter did approach. Fire was also used to cook and to prepare our food.

Then a rival "light" appeared on this earth in 1879 when Thomas Edison invented the light bulb using electricity and a carbon filament in an oxygen-free bulb that glowed at high temperatures – emitting again such mysterious waves - and gave light for about forty hours. This invention was soon perfected to result in our now known light bulb which started to light up the homes and cities and darkness could be converted into light with the push of a switch.

In addition, some of the first primitive organisms like fireflies and some fish living in deep, dark waters started to create their own sources of light called bioluminescence. They used it and still use it to communicate with each other like finding a mate or to catch prey.

The importance of the sun and "light" in human life was recognized quite early since the first civilizations arose (about 3000 BCE). People realized that our life and that of fruits and crops and animals depended on the sun. These civilizations believed in one or in many sun gods which were revered and worshipped. Most of these sun deities were male while the moon was associated more often with female deities. In Egyptian mythology, the sun god had to pass through darkness and had to defeat the god of darkness each day in order to re-appear the next morning. The Sun God in Hinduism received immense worship and was associated with bringing light to mankind and with life per se. Helios was the sun god of the Greeks who drove the sun across the sky from east to west in a golden chariot and the sun would then move back across the ocean to its origin. The Aztecs were fascinated with the sun god who demanded human sacrifices (and it has been estimated that about 10 000 victims were sacrificed each year). In the Christian religion, the importance of light was also recognized in that God created light on the very first day of creation of the world with the bible telling us: Let there be light (Of course, if the bible would have been written to day, the words would have been: Let there be special waves which human eyes and brains can convert into light and sight – and only after the first humans and animals with eyes and brains were created did light and sight then finally appear). The divine nature of light was the common belief for most civilizations for thousands of years.

Soon scholars started to look at "light" more closely including some of their daily experiences with light. One of the first experience must have been when people were looking in still water and seeing their faces and later on when looking at a shiny surface and again seeing their faces or other objects. It became also known quite early that the water or surface had to be plane to see an image and that an uneven surface would distort the image. This became known as reflection. Reflection was first studied extensively by the Greek scholar Euclid (about 300 BCE) using strict geometry. He found already that the incoming and outgoing angle of light were the same (A=B) which is still the fundamental law of reflection today.

He also showed geometrically how we see ourselves in a mirror. Reflection is not only important how we see each other in a mirror but for vision in general. If objects would not reflect light waves from our surroundings into our eyes we would not be able to see them. In addition, reflection is used in science and technology and in many medical instruments and devices including those used in ophthalmology.

Soon another phenomenon was investigated which must also have been observed since ancient times. This was when looking at a stick partly immersed in water. The stick seems to show a bend or seems to be broken where it entered the water. This became known as refraction. Refraction is the bending of light when it passes from one medium (e.g. air) into a denser medium (e.g. water) except when it enters this medium perpendicularly.

One of the first who applied mathematics to refraction was the Roman/Greek scholar Ptolemy in about 140 CE. He had observed through his astronomical studies that light from the sun and the stars would be refracted through the atmosphere. He found a simple equation to calculate the path of light outside and in the water. He described an experiment where he placed a coin in an empty metal jar which could not be seen from the outside (arrow shows our path of vision in the empty jar). Then he filled the jar partly with water and the coin could be seen because the light (two arrows) did bent or refract the light to the coin:

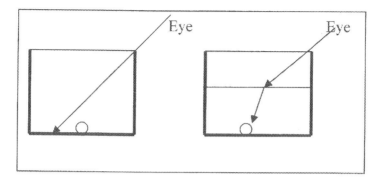

Figure 26

He also looked at refraction in the earth's atmosphere and assumed that light rays must bend as they pass from thinner to denser air and concluded that we will not see celestial bodies where they actually are. This is, of course, true. This law of refraction was then rediscovered and refined later on by the English scholar Snell in 1621. Refraction makes our vision possible by focusing objects through the cornea and lens exactly on the retina. Refraction allows us to correct vision problems through eye glasses or contact lenses, Lasik surgery and the implantation of intraocular lenses after cataract surgery.

The next property of light scholars became interested in was its speed or how fast "light" would travel. It was most likely recognized early on that the moment the sun appeared on the horizon darkness disappeared rapidly and it became light very quickly. Light must have travelled very fast through space to light and warm the earth, to make us do our daily chores right after sunrise and to allow the plants to grow. Greek scholars pondered this question and most – although not all - agreed that light had infinite speed. Looking at the sun which is very far away it can nevertheless be seen instantaneously – thus, light must travel at infinite speed. This was the common belief until the early middle ages.

Some scholars in the early middle ages then proposed that light might actually have a finite albeit very fast speed. One of the first scholars who tried to measure the speed of light was Galileo (1564-1642). But with the crude time pieces available at this time – he used most likely a water clock –- he was unable to come to a firm result. He concluded that light must travel very fast (although mechanical clocks were available at this time but they still were quite inaccurate and were massive and mostly used for cathedrals – such a clock was installed in the cathedral of Salisbury in England in 1386 and is still working today with its original mechanism). In 1676 the Danish scholar Ole Christensen Roemer made the first measurement of the speed of light by observing a moon of Jupiter. He noticed that the time which elapsed between eclipses of this moon by Jupiter became shorter as Earth moved closer to Jupiter and became longer as Earth and Jupiter moved farther apart. He reasoned that – since the moon's circle was constant – the light must have traveled different distances from Jupiter to earth from these two locations – one closer and one farther away from earth. Based on this observation he concluded that light traveled at about 225 000 km/sec (which was astoundingly close to its actual speed considering the primitive instruments available at this time). Later on, scholars used more refined techniques and improved the value to be between 297 000 and 303 000 km/sec. Further refinements brought the speed of light in a vacuum to its now accepted value - 299,792,458 meters per second (or roughly 300 000 km/sec). According to Einstein's theory of relativity nothing could move faster because this would require an infinite amount of energy and would mean that a person moving faster than light would theoretically arrive at a destination before leaving it. Interestingly, a team of researchers from the Ecole Polytechnique in Lausanne (EPFL) claimed recently that they successfully demonstrated, for the first time, that it is possible to actually speed light up in certain optical devices past the currently accepted maximal speed. This might mean that physicists will have to revise Einstein's special theory of relativity. It has also been suggested that at the beginning of the universe or the BIG Bang, the explosion occurred faster than the 299,792,458 meters per second. The speed of light is of no major consequence in our daily lives. Nevertheless, when we see a sun just setting we have to be aware of the fact that the sun already had set for about 8 minutes (the time it takes light to travel from the sun to the earth). Of course, these aberrations become enormous when we consider the vastness of the universe and trying to locate a star in the telescope which is billions of miles away.

Nobody, however, was really concerned with the physical nature or what light actually is until up to about 1650. Light was taken for granted and ancient scholars looked at it as a divine gift and only few ventured an explanation as to its nature. One was Lucretius who wrote in *On the nature of the Universe* (55 CE) " *The light and heat of the sun; these are composed of minute atoms which, when they are shoved off, lose no time in shooting right across the interspace of air in the direction imparted by the shove*". But this was not readily accepted and in the western medieval ages since light was firmly believed to be of a divine nature – God had created light and only God would know what light is. The renowned English scholar Grosseteste stated around 1200 that God is light and light would bring us closer to God. A more naturalistic explanation was offered by Descartes (1596-1650) who proposed that we see an object in that immaterial impulses would be traveling from this object through a medium (e.g. air) to our eyes which would then be felt (like we would feel an object through a stick on our hands). The real first clue based on experimental evidence and not speculation was provided by the English scholar and physicist Isaac Newton (1642-1727) who is often better known as the discoverer of gravity due to an alleged apple falling on his head. In around 1660 CE he experimented with light and passed a beam of light through a prism (a triangular shaped piece of crystal). To his amazement, he saw white light entering the crystal but a spectrum of colors emerging from the opposite side. These colors – as mentioned before- were <u>r</u>ed, <u>o</u>range, <u>y</u>ellow, <u>g</u>reen, <u>b</u>lue, <u>i</u>ndigo and <u>v</u>iolet (to be remembered as <u>Roy G. Biv</u> or <u>R</u>ichard <u>o</u>f <u>Y</u>ork <u>g</u>ave <u>b</u>attle <u>i</u>n <u>v</u>ain). If a second prism was then positioned in such a way as to catch the different colors they would combine and white light would leave the second prism. Of course, rainbows with these colors had been seen since ancient times but their nature was never explored and contributed to supernatural phenomena. Newton now posited for the first time a scientific explanation of the nature of light we see in that white light was actually a combination of the seven individual colors and would consist of little particles or corpuscles which would travel from the object through the environment to the eye. The first scientific theory of light – the corpuscular theory had arrived. But not completely – Newton was a very religious person and firmly believed that all earthly physics and natural events including light were under the influence and supervision of God. The corpuscular theory can be pictured below in that from the object O light particles (.) would be emitted and would travel to our eye (Eye) where they would be felt:

O .... Eye

This corpuscular theory of light was soon challenged by the Dutch scholar Christiaan Huygens in about 1680 who also experimented with light and performed experiments which could only be explained if light was a wave and not a particle. However, his light waves were still longitudinal traveling into one direction (or if an object would be placed on such a wave it would be carried into this direction). The scholars at this time were now divided into two camps but the majority favored Newton's theory due to his outstanding reputation. However, the Jesuit priest, mathematician and physicist Grimaldi had already shown around 1650 that light is bend around edges of opaque objects or a light shining on this object will produce a dark shadow with some very light shadow at its edges (a phenomenon called diffraction). This phenomenon cannot be explained by particles which would pass straight along the edges without casting a shadow. Waves, however, can be bent on edges and these bent rays form the light shadow. Finally, the English physician and scholar Young performed the crucial experiment in about 1810 which demonstrated that light was indeed a wave. He let sunlight shine through a tiny hole and then held edgewise a very thin card into the beam to split it in two parts. The projection of the split screen revealed a pattern of light and dark lines. He also let light shine through two pinholes and observed the same pattern. These findings could not be explained by the corpuscular theory but can be explained by the wave theory where waves were bent or deflected from the edges and would overlap. Waves could then augment (crests of two waves would meet) showing light spots or cancel each other (crest of one wave would meet the trough of another wave) showing dark spots. This is referred to as interference. With these experiments on diffraction and interference the nature of light was now firmly established as a wave although these waves were still thought to travel longitudinal and not up and down. In this case, particles move into one direction (e.g. left to right) and bunch together and spread out to be bunched together again and to be spread out and so forth (here, a wave length is from one point of highest density to the next point of highest density).

But there was still a problem – if there were waves there must be something which would move (like waves in the water where water molecules would move). To find a solution, an invisible and matterless substance called "ether" (not the ether we know from chemistry) was postulated which would be the medium which would create and propagate the light waves (in a push-like matter). In 1810, experiments by Malus, Arago and Fresnel showed that light waves were actually vertical or moving up and down in all directions. These scholars noticed that the reflections of the setting sun on a crystal changed intensity depending on how the crystal was rotated (a phenomenon later called polarization). Passing light through different crystals they found that light would pass either through or not depended on the rotation of these crystals. They theorized that light was made of transverse waves changing directions very fast. This can be visualized schematically if light would oscillate horizontally and vertically (although it does it in all direction in nature) and if this schematic light would pass through an object with a very small horizontal slit (removing all "waves" except the horizontal waves), light could still be seen passing through the slit. But if a second object with a vertical small slit would by placed behind, no light would be seen because the vertical "waves " cannot pass through the horizontal slit:

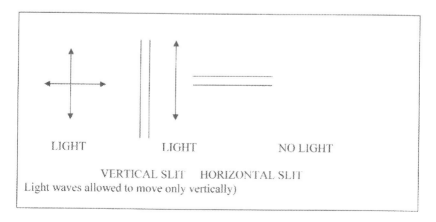

LIGHT   LIGHT   NO LIGHT

VERTICAL SLIT   HORIZONTAL SLIT
Light waves allowed to move only vertically)

Figure 27

Light was now accepted by scientists to consist of vertical waves changing direction very rapidly. Polarized sun glasses use this principle. Light reflects from surfaces in all directions which can cause a glare or an annoying intensity of light. Polarized sun glasses filter the light – like the light has to go through a slit – and remove all of those waves which do not pass through this "slit". This reduces the amount of waves reaching the eye and we experience less glare.

Up to this point light consisted of the seven spectral colors. However, in 1800 Herschel found that there is invisible light beyond red which he called infrared light and in 1801 Ritter found that there is invisible light beyond blue which he called chemical light and which we now refer to as ultraviolet light. These waves can not be seen be our eyes but can only be detected by physical instruments. Thus, the spectrum of light began to expand and it now has expanded even further beyond infrared and ultraviolet waves.

But the exact nature of these mysterious waves was still unknown. This changed when the Scottish physicist James Clark Maxwell (about 1850) posited through brilliant mathematical deductions and equations that light waves were actually invisible electromagnetic waves. His conclusion was based on the discoveries of two previous scientists. This is another instance, how knowledge from history promotes new ideas. In 1820 the Danish professor Oersted had found that an electrical current would deflect a close by compass needle (held at right angle to the electrical wire) and deduced that electrical currents could cause a magnetic field. In 1831, the English Scientist Faraday inspired by this experiment tried the opposite: he moved a magnet through a coiled wire and created an electrical current. These discoveries are being used to day to create our electricity in electrical generators–rotating magnets inside electrical wires - and to drive electromotors – rotating electrical wires inside a magnet. Maxwell now connected these two events through several mathematical equations which described the physical nature of these "electromagnetic" waves moving through the hypothetical ether. He then calculated the speed of these waves and found them to be about 300 000 km/sec. This number reminded him of another number, namely the speed of light as it had been calculated before.

This previous knowledge let him to conclude that light consists of electromagnetic waves. He wrote" *The velocity of transverse undulations (waves) in our hypothetical medium ---agrees so exactly with the velocity of light -----that we can scarcely avoid the inference that light consists in the transverse undulations (waves) of the same medium which is the cause of electric and magnetic phenomenon.*" Individual colors were then just electromagnetic waves of different wave lengths. He later on abandoned the idea that a hypothetical ether was necessary for the transmission of the waves which was experimentally proven to be correct later on by other scientists. The actual existence of these electromagnetic waves was shown by the German physicist Heinrich Hertz (about 1880) who experimentally demonstrated the existence of electromagnetic waves in the laboratory by observing an electric spark each time an electromagnetic wave would be received by a metallic object.

Then an unexpected and surprising event occurred. The German physicist Max Planck (around 1900) showed that light energy is emitted and absorbed in distinct minute chunks or units or quanta or particles and Einstein finally explained mathematically the existence of these now called photons (for which he received the Nobel prize in 1921). Thus, light now seemed to consist again of distinct particles which were called photons. What was so clear before became now again complex: is light a wave or a photon (a particle)? Here, Einstein showed that light actually could consist of either particles or waves depending on the circumstances and conditions and how we look at it. However, this is a pure theoretical, mathematical and physical problem and for most optical and physiological considerations we need to know that light can be considered a wave.

Although electrical waves and magnetic fields can not be seen, their relationship can perhaps be visualized as shown below with the light gray waves representing an electrical wave and the perpendicular dark waves the magnetic field:

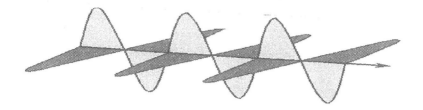

Figure 28

The nature and properties of these electromagnetic waves are very important because they are the basis of our vision. The nature of these waves and their interactions with the photosensitive cells in our eyes explains how we see in general, how we see colors and can help in the future to perhaps cure vision problems by implanting chips into the eye which respond selectively to these waves.

While the physical nature of light has now almost deciphered (details still need to be ironed out by theoretical physicists) we should not forget the other perhaps non-physical side of "light". The German playwright and scientist von Goethe published what was intuitively known for centuries that light and its colors also had an emotional component and wrote around 1800: *"Colors contain a living force – and whenever a human sees a color he experiences delight and joy"* (and he might be called the father of color psychology). We all know how colors affect our emotions in that certain colors are found pleasant and soothing while others are found appalling and depressing.

Light also affects our well being in that prolonged darkness like the winters in the very northern countries leads to an increased risk of suicide and some people suffer from depression in our areas during the winter months which can be cured by light exposure.

Eye and Brain. Before the complex processes involving vision can be deciphered, the anatomy of the eye and of the brain must be known and the next paragraphs will deal with the histories of the anatomy or structure of the human eye and the brain and their functions as they slowly developed over the last 3000 years. As described in some detail in the chapter "How animals do see" it all started out with single cells which finally developed into human eyes and brains making it possible for us to see. Here, we will only deal with the history of the human eye and brain and how their structures and functions were discovered.

Ancient people, of course, knew that we possessed two eyes but their structure and function was unknown unless some unfortunate people lost part or all of their vision and could not see anymore. Punishment for certain crimes in some of these early civilizations was "blinding" the offender. In contrast, people born blind were often revered as specially blessed by the Gods and Homer, the Greek story teller of the Trojan War, was blind. The oldest legal document, the code of Hammurabi (Mesopotamia) written around 1700 BCE mentions the importance of the human eye: "*If a physician ---- opens a tumor with the operating knife, and cuts out the eye, his hands shall be cut off*". The Old Testament speaks about: an eye for an eye. However, among the ancient civilizations like the Sumerians, Indians, Persians or Egyptians only the Greek seemed to have had a scientific interest in the eye and its structure and function. They were the first scholars who studied and depicted the anatomy of the eye as the seat of vision more closely. This was no easy task because the eye usually collapses if it is removed from the head and cut. They described a transparent membrane (cornea) and an opaque membrane (sclera) with a hole in the middle (pupil). These two layers enclosed a fluid substance (viscous). The eye was regarded as the principle site of vision and a tube leading from the eye to the brain allowed the movement of a "visual" substance from the brain into the eye (the tube was most likely the optic nerve but not recognized as such). The eye according to Democritus around 450 BCE looked like this:

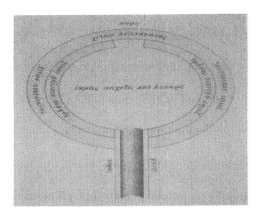

Figure 29

Later on, most likely based on the dissection of animal eyes, three layers were recognized. The retina was not mentioned. The ocular fluid was considered to be uniform and the lens was thought to form after death by solidification of fluid through exposure to air.

During this time, physicians and scholars also studied the brain. Before, prehistoric people already knew that the skull and its inside had some importance since skulls with holes from these times were found. Apparently these holes were made by scraping (called trepanation) away the bone with a sharp stone until the brain could be seen. Surprisingly, people must have survived this procedure because the rim of the holes of some of these skulls showed new bone growth. Why this was done is unknown but it is assumed that people were perhaps plagued by terrific headaches which were thought to be caused by an evil demon trapped inside the skull. The remedy, of course, would then be to drill a hole through the skull through which the demon could escape. Interestingly, this was performed in different areas of the world which were not connected to each other indicating that this practice must have developed independently. It was also still performed in Africa by certain tribes until about 1970. Movie clips from these later trepanations showed the "patient" sitting quietly while the "surgeon" scraped away the bone (which is extremely painful) until the brain could be seen. The "surgeon" would then pour some water over the wound from a dish from which a goat had satisfied its thirst before (the goat was actually the fee for the operation) and finally bandaged the opening with plant leaves. The patient survived and it was found out later that this was actually her third trepanation. The picture below shows an ancient trephined skull:

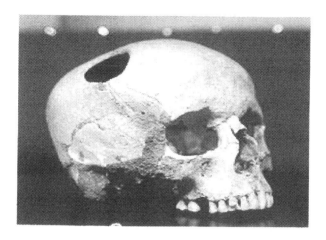

Figure 30

It can be seen that the edges of the hole are quite smooth indicating that this individual must have survived the operation and new bone had formed over the next years.

Again, only the Greek scholars among all the ancient scholars also thought about the brain. The brain assumed two different functions around 400 BCE. Alcmaeon, one of the first ancient Greek philosophers, proposed that the brain was the organ of thought and that the nerves leaving the eye are light-bearing paths to and from the brain. In contrast, Aristotle (384-322 BCE) posited that the organ of thought and emotions was the heart and the brain functioned only as an accessory organ to regulate heat and cool the body. Due to the importance of Aristotle his theory prevailed for some time. It has even survived into modern times where we still use expressions like: I love you with all my heart or I know this by heart. The Greek scholars Herophiles and Erasistratus (around 300 BCE) were among the first to dissect human bodies and the brain. They distinguished the cerebrum (larger portion) from the cerebellum (smaller portion) and suggested that the ventricles or cavities in the brain were the actual seat of intelligence. They identified the nerves and thought of them as tubes through which a "special fluid" or "animal spirit" would flow. They also noted the difference between motor nerves (those concerned with motion) and sensory nerves (those related to sensation including vision).

The ancient Egyptians – like Aristotle in Greece - believed that the heart is the most important part of the body and the seat of good and evil. Thus, the heart was carefully preserved during the embalming process while the brain was extracted from the skull through the nose and discarded as an unimportant organ during mummification.

During the Roman Empire, physicians and scholars most notably Galen (about 175 CE) and Celsus (about 200 CE) continued to study the eye and brain. They reviewed the existing Greek literature, compiled its knowledge, added their own experiments, observations and theories and published their works. For the eye, they added the lens (now present in the living eye which previously had been thought to be solidification due to death), the conjunctiva as an extra membrane, the distinct retina (the name derived from the Greek word for "fishnet" like structure) and the optic nerve which was thought to be still hollow. The tubes from each eye would then fuse at the chiasm in the brain. However, it was stated that the optic nerve *"which comes from the right side of the brain goes to the right eye, and the nerve which comes from the left side goes to the left eye"* which is only partially true for humans (and might have derived from experiments with birds where this indeed is the case). The anatomy of the eye according to Galen about 150 CE had improved markedly and looked like this:

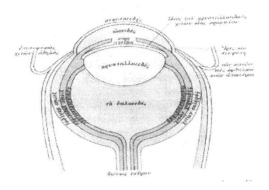

Figure 31

Galen disagreed with Aristotle and concluded that the brain was the seat of the "animal soul" (meaning mind and it would also form sperms in men). He wrote that the ventricles (cavities in the brain) were the receptacles for this "soul". They were formed to become the place for our sensory, motor and cognitive functions. Later, they were classified as the "impressiva" which was the first cavity and which gathered information from all the senses. It then passes the information to the second one "sensus communis" where the information was processed and executed. The third one was "memoria" where the information would be remembered. This was the common perception for the next 1500 years and the three chambers are beautifully depicted by Leonardo da Vinci about 1500.

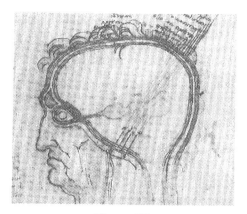

Figure 32

Galen also preached that the four humors in our body – which were thought by the ancient Greeks to be blood, phlegm and yellow and black bile - would affect the brain and the temperament of the person. A balance among the humors provided bodily as well as mental health and an imbalance of any of them caused bodily and mental illness.

Until about 1500, scholars in the western world who were mostly well educated monks or priests relied solely on the writings of ancient scholars like Galen and the preaching of the Church. They did little if any scholarly work themselves. Eyes and the brain were created by God and only God did know how they were constructed and how they worked. It was permissible to study and explore nature but just to understand how wonderfully God had created our world. Nature was not of interest per se but was a way to better understand God and to lead us to our creator.

While knowledge about the eye and brain (as well as other bodily organs) stagnated during this time in the Western world and while the old Greek writings were largely ignored and forgotten, Islamic scholars of the then mighty Islamic nation which around 800 CE covered an area from the East over Africa to Spain collected the old Greek books and translated them into Arabic. This was a tremendous and rewarding deed because many of the old Greek writings were forgotten and started to become lost. Today we know of their contents in many cases only through their translations and preservation into the Arabic language. At first, Arabic scholars contributed little to the knowledge of the anatomy of the eye and brain. Later on, these scholars and physicians started their own investigations and studies of the brain. They developed new experimental approaches to understand the workings of the mind and established what one might call to-day the field of psychology. Among other investigations, these scholars were very much interested in dreams and their interpretations. Avicenna who lived around 1000 CE was one of the first scholars to divide human perception into the five senses of hearing, seeing, feeling, smelling and tasting. He dissected the brain and discovered certain distinct sub-structures. In addition, they also became the leading physicians and scholars during this time and established many educational centers and libraries throughout the Arabic nation. Bagdad became the center of medical and intellectual knowledge and activity. Unfortunately for medicine and science, scientific and medical activities started to decline rapidly after the 12th century due to a break-up of the Islamic Empire, pressure from the outside world both from the west (crusades!) and Mongolia (the Mongols sacked Bagdad and destroyed many of the precious writings and books) and a rise in Islamic theology which replaced scientific and medical studies with religious views.

Around 1500, a change occurred in the western world which is called the Renaissance. Scholars started to re-discover the old Greek writings, to collect the few remaining old Greek books and to translate others from Arabic into Latin. The dominance of the Catholic Church began to erode due to the emergence of various protestant religions and the expansion of the world by the discovery of the Americas. Physicians and scholars broke slowly away from the teachings of Galen and started their own independent research and investigations. Physicians would now more aggressively dissect the human body including the eye and the brain - often in conflict with the Church and worldly authorities who forbade dissections. Early physicians had to obtain bodies legally from executed criminals and if this supply dwindled they had to rob graves by themselves or by hiring often poor and desperate men (thus, physicians were referred to as "grave robbers"). Dissecting such partly decomposed bodies with their horrendous smell was indeed a courageous undertaking perhaps somewhat tolerable in the winter months (when most dissections indeed took place) but almost unbearable in the hot summer days. Of interest is that one of the first who dissected the human body – mostly for his artistic work but also to satisfy his own anatomical and scientific curiosity – was the painter, sculptor, architect, inventor and scientist Leonardo da Vinci around 1500. He made elaborate and meticulous drawings of individual body parts. He studied the eye which is difficult to dissect in that he encased it in egg white and then boiled it so that it would solidify for easier cutting. Unfortunately, he recorded his findings only in his numerous note books but never made them public. They were only found later and translated in many languages. The German Jesuit priest and natural philosopher Christoph Scheiner (around 1600) discovered that the optic nerve would not leave the eye opposite the pupil but sideways towards the nose. Thus, at this time most major anatomical structures of the eye (except for the ciliary body) were known to scientists and physicians.

Similarly, the gross anatomy of the brain became known and it was realized that the brain size and mass increased as one went up the evolutionary ladder – humans had the largest brain in the animal kingdom (based on body weight). But this gross anatomy was now investigated in more detail. These investigations began with the Belgian physician and anatomist Andreas Vesalius who methodically and systematically dissected human bodies in 1550 but also had an artist make accurate and elaborate drawings of the body and its individual organs and parts. He soon published an extensive book with beautiful and detailed pictures of the human anatomy. He also published a more exact picture of the brain and disputed the assumption that the mental functions are situated in the ventricles but suggested them to occur in the matter of the brain per se – since animals have ventricles but cannot reason like humans.

Descartes – known for his famous saying: cogito ergo sum or I think therefore I am – still believed in the importance of the ventricles but introduced in addition the pineal body in about 1625 as the "*rational soul* " (meaning mind – wisely he left the religious soul out of his design and in the hands of the Church) which he proposed to be the chief engineer of the brain exerting over-all control of our brain activities. He also introduced the dual system of the material brain and the immaterial mind which is still being debated today (whereas it is unclear how an immaterial mind can interact with a material brain and vise versa). From now on physicians studied the brain more extensively and a number of books describing the anatomy of the brain were published, for instance, by the English physician Thomas Willis (1664) and the Danish anatomist Nicolaus Steno (1669). Both criticized Galen in general as well as in his description of the brain and Steno wrote that "*animal spirits*" were "*words without any meaning.*" These studies squarely placed our mental functions into the brain and later into the cortex.

Up to this time, the naked eye was the only instrument to study the anatomy of the eye, nerves and brain although some scholars might have used the magnifying glass which was already known at this time under the name of "*reading stone*". This changed with the discovery of the microscope. The early credit for inventing the microscope might have to go to Hans and Zacharias Janssen in Holland around 1600 who made a simple microscope consisting of a tube and some lenses. But the first to examine biological material in greater detail with the microscope was Anton van Leeuwenhoek in about 1660. He was a merchant in Delft, Holland, who developed an interest in this newly discovered device and in biology and became a self-made biologist. He refined the microscope further (keeping its individual constructions a secret) and studied and published microscopic pictures of biological specimens (including little "creatures" he found swimming in stale water which were never seen before and which he called "animalcules"), blood vessels and red blood cells. He also examined animal eyes and discovered some of its finer structures unknown up to this time. This was followed by Robert Hooke in about 1680, British scientist and inventor, who refined the microscope even further and discovered certain small and repeating structures when examining samples of cork. He named these small structures which occur in all biological materials: cells – and this word is still being used today - and they were soon recognized as the smallest anatomical units of all organisms.

Using better and more efficient designed microscopes, special cells in the retina were discovered in the 1830s by German Scholars which later on were identified as rods and cones. In 1850 it was found that cones were the color receptors while the rods were very light sensitive but did not respond to colors. In 1850 the ciliary body in the eye was discovered by the German physician Bruecke and the English physician Bowman and the lens was now suspended with zonules between this muscle. It was not necessary anymore to posit that the lens was a muscle which would change its curvature by itself but this job was now done by the ciliary body. During these times, the nerve cells of the retina were also discovered and could now be divided roughly into four groups such as ganglion cells, amacrine cells, bipolar cells and horizontal cells. At this time the gross structure of the eye was known and the eye now consisted of its major components such as the three membranes, cornea, anterior chamber (aqueous humor), iris with pupil, the ciliary body with the lens inside a capsule suspended by the zonules, the vitreous (vitreous humor) and retina consisting of two kinds of photosensitive cells (cones, rods) and four different nerve cells one of which could extend into the optic nerve radiating towards the brain.

The discovery of the electron microscope in 1940 allowed scientists to obtain even finer details of all of the ocular structures. Now the details of the eye including the retina with its photosensitive cells and nerve cells were known and only residual details have still to be ironed out in the future.

The understanding of the finer aspects of the anatomy and in particular the functioning of the brain also began to unravel after the discovery of the microscope which allowed scientists to see individual nerve cells. However, this took a slower course. The first nerve cells were apparently seen by Ehrenberg in 1833 and later by Purkinje and the Italian Golgi developed a stain in 1873 which selectively stained nerve cells so that they could be visualized under the microscope. Again, the electron microscope allowed an even closer look at the innermost details of the brain including the blood vessels and neurons (plus supporting cells such as glia cells). In 1954, the first pictures were developed showing vesicles or little packages within neurons containing neurotransmitters.

As the anatomy of the brain became more and more known, the function of a nerve was still highly speculative. Up to the end of the 18th century, nerves were still considered hollow tubes filled with special fluids or 'animal spirits". This changed with the Italian scholar Luigi Galvani who observed during his experiments in 1775 that frog legs would twitch when exposed to electricity and posited that the nerves make the muscle move via an "*animal electricity*" (to set it aside from other known types of electricity like static electricity or lightning). He replaced the ancient view of a special nerve fluid as the controlling function of the nerves with electricity. Later on, the term "animal electricity" was abandoned since all electricities were shown to be alike. Nevertheless, he proved that our nerves used electricity to do their jobs in making us see, move, feel and think. Nerves conducted electricity which then allows them to communicate with each other and which makes our muscles contract. In the case of our eyes, electrical activity (now referred to as nerve impulses) conducts the information from the eyes through the optic nerve to the various brain areas.

But how did this electricity in our nerves originate or what caused it to move along neurons? The answer to this question had to wait until around 1950 when the English physiologists/pharmacologists Huxley, Hodgkin, Katz and Eccles found while investigating the activity of a nerve cell of the squid (which is particularly large) that electrically charged sodium and potassium particles (called ions) would flow in and out of this nerve. They posited these movements of the electrically charged particles to be the cause of the electrical currents occurring in all neurons. This was confirmed by other experiments to be indeed so. Now the origin and nature of a nerve impulse was established.

But there was still a problem. Anatomical studies had shown that nerves do not connect directly to other nerves or other structures in the body like muscles. In all these cases, there is a small gap between them called a synapse. How could nerves then activate other nerves or control muscles? Did electricity jump over this gap as proposed by some scientists? The final answer was provided by an experiment performed by Loewi, a German pharmacologist, who worked in Austria. In the 1920s, he stimulated a special nerve leading to the isolated heart of a frog beating in a fluid filled glass jar (yes, hearts can beat outside the body when some fluid is forced into them). This nerve was known to slow the heart (vagus nerve) and indeed it did do so in this experiment. But then he transferred some of the fluid from this jar to another, second isolated heart in another jar – and he found it would also slow the beating of this heart as well. The only way the fluid from the first heart could slow the second heart was that a chemical must have been released from the stimulated nerve of the first heart preparation which was still present in the fluid when applied to the second heart. This chemical was later on identified by the English physiologist/pharmacologist Dale to be acetylcholine which directly applied to the heart would indeed slow the heart beat or it would when applied to a muscle cause it to contract. Later on, other such chemicals were found which would also initiate nerve impulses or contract muscles. They are now called neurotransmitters. A neurotransmitter is usually released from one nerve cell and when binding to an adjacent nerve cell will initiate a nerve impulse in this neuron or when binding to a muscle will make it to contract. Now the communication between a nerve and a nerve or a nerve and a muscle was established to be chemical in nature and is now referred to as neurotransmission.

Now the anatomy and basic neuronal processes of the brain were known – but what about the inner workings of the brain. How and where, for instance, do we feel, think, control our muscles and, in this case, see. Does this occur all over the brain or are there special areas involved for these special tasks as suggested by previous scholars but never been demonstrated. Here, head injuries obtained by accidents or in war times, strokes and later on brain surgery helped us to begin to understand the functions of the brain and to identify certain crucial areas. It was an accident in1848 which showed that the brain and one part in particular would play a significant role in our mental activities, functions and behavior. Phineas Gage was a railroad worker with a fine work record and a very pleasant and nice personality. During an explosion an iron rod went through his head and destroyed his frontal brain lobe but – miraculously - he survived and recovered. However, he showed marked personality changes after his recovery in that he now became lazy, combative and aggressive and could not hold a job. Around 1860, the French physician Paul Broca had a patient with severe speech problems. When he autopsied him later on he found damage to one particular area in the brain which is now referred to as Brocas area and which is involved in the regulation of proper speech. The Canadian neurosurgeon Wilder Penfield performed extensive brain surgeries on patients while being conscious during the 1940s and 1950s (although the brain experiences the pain from all sites of the body, it feels no pain itself and a needle can be inserted into the brain without the patient experiencing any pain). He stimulated then specific regions of the brains of his patients with an electrode and asked them what they felt. All kinds of sensations, images and even memories were elicited. It was also soon discovered that certain areas of the brain correlated with sensations from various body parts and a theoretical "sensory homunculus" could be constructed along the brain where a certain area would correspond to a certain body part.

However, it was also quickly discovered that these specific areas while performing specific tasks do not work in isolation but need the assistance of other areas as well. Damage to a certain area in the brain was found, for instance, to interfere with a complete vision task by, for example, disconnecting seeing from comprehending. Such an individual will clearly see a face which could be a familiar one or even his own face but will not know whose face it is. Also, the brain is very adapted to compensate for damage to one area. If Brocas area is damaged quickly, speech difficulties will ensue. If a slow growing tumor destroys this area gradually, no problems may arise because other areas will then slowly assume the speech tasks.

Today with magnetic resonance imaging (MRI) we can look at the brain and its finer details without opening the skull in the living person and with positron emission tomography (PET) we can even observe those brain areas which will become active during certain mental activities because they will light up on a screen.

Although the size of the human brain is important it is not the sole determining factor. The brain of Albert Einstein was average in size and weight (although it showed an enlarged area for abstract thinking at the cost of a reduced area for speech which most likely accounted for his delayed speaking as a child). What seems to be of most importance for our mental functions is not brain size but the number of neuronal networks and circuits it contains. This is similar to a computer chip - it is not the size of the chip in a computer which gives it its power but the number of bytes it contains. Today's research is now concerned to decipher how the electrical activity of these networks and circuits in our brains is converted to form our cognition, our thoughts, our feelings, our memories and, of course, our visual images.

Vision. As the knowledge of the nature of light and the anatomy of the eyes, nerves and brain slowly developed over the last 2500 years, so did our knowledge about the visual processes. Only this information allowed scholars to finally figure out how our eyes and brains would interact with the electromagnetic waves coming from our environment and cause us to see our world.

Ancient people were well aware that they could see and must have been distressed if vision declined or was lost. However, only the ancient Greek again pondered and theorized about how we actually see. Democritus about 450 BCE and Epicurus about 300 BCE thought that extremely thin slices or images of worldly objects would continuously slough off from these objects, travel to our eyes and were then seen. This became known as the intromission theory. Unfortunately, they could not explain how slices of a very large object could enter our smaller eyes or why objects would not become smaller over time if they loose these slices continuously. In contrast, Alcmaeon and Euclid about 350 BCE assumed that there is some sort of 'internal fire' in our eyes –like an internal lantern - which would be issued from our eyes. This "fire" would seek the objects in the environment and, when found, would 'feel' these objects (similar to touch) and transmit their findings back to our eyes. This became known as the extramission theory. Again, they could not explain why we then could not see in darkness if we would send out this "fire" or how our internal "fire" could reach the sun which is so far away. It was Aristotle (about 350 BCE) who supplied us with a slightly different theory. He emphasized light and color and wrote: *"what is visible, is color"* and " *color is not visible without light"*. He thought that light would come from the color of the object and would alter the "medium" (or air) between the object itself and the viewer's eye. This alteration of the medium was thought to be felt by the eye allowing the object to be seen. He based his theory on the importance of the medium between the object and eye and that an object held very close to the eye can not be seen. He also warned that we can easily be perceived by our senses *"the sun appears only a foot in diameter but we are convinced that it is larger"*. Basically, the seat of vision was thought by all scholars to be in the eyes (in general) and the two theories of vision – the intromission (light from objects) and extramission (light from eyes) theory - would now be debated by scholars for the next 1500 years with the extramission theory being dominant during this time.

Euclid around 350 BCE was the first who tried to use geometry to explain how we see objects (and it will be shown later on that geometry indeed plays a major role in deciphering the optical part of our visual process). He tried -among other explanations - to demonstrate why we see the same object larger or smaller depending on its distance from the eye. He showed geometrically – using the extramission theory - *"that things seen under a larger angle appear larger, those under a smaller angle appear smaller"* (which is still valid today):

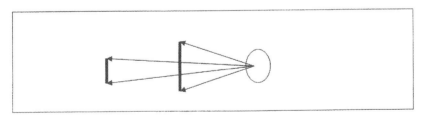

Figure 33

The extramission theory – light being emitted from the eyes - was then promoted by the Roman scholars like Galen and Ptolemy (CE 100-170) and became the dominant theory in the West in the early medieval ages. Ptolemy argued that vision consisted of three phases. The first phase is physical in nature and consists of a visual flux originating in the body's governing facility (brain), moving into the eyes and leaving the eyes in form of a cone with the apex in the eye. The second phase is when the visual flux or rays like tentacles "feel" the object which must be compact and illuminated and have color. This gives a certain "passion" to the visual flux which conveys the object's physical shapes and properties to the eye. During the third phase the "feeling" is now converted in the eyes (this is somewhat unclear) into the object as it exists in space.

Islamic scholars who dominated the scientific and medical disciplines in the early medieval ages also debated the two theories of extra- and intromission and the intromission theory finally became dominant – mostly based on the work and writings of the Arabic scholar Alhazen (about 1000 CE). He argued if one looks at the sun, the eyes hurt – this would not happen if light originates from the eyes to reach the sun but only if light – in this case too much light – originated from the sun and would reach the eye.

During the early and middle medieval ages in the western world, the works of Galen and Ptolemy still dominated the knowledge on vision. It was thought that *"the crystalline lens is the principal instrument of vision, a fact clearly proved by what physicians call cataracts, which lie between the crystalline humor* (lens) *and the cornea and interfere with vision until they are couched* "(like a curtain before the lens which would be pushed down during couching and the lens would receive light again – see later under ocular medicine). This changed during the renaissance when scholars accepted the intromission theory and started again to study geometrically our visual processes. The German scholar and royal mathematician Johannes Kepler (around 1600) who is best known for his discovery of the ways the planets circle around the earth also was interested in vision and applied geometry to visual problems. He found out that the lens (still thought to be the site of vision at this time) was just an optical device and its purpose was to project a precise image of an object accurately onto the retina. The retina now became the important part of the eye where a picture was actually received. He also stated that this image on the retina was upside down and right-left side reversed – which provoked a lot of criticism and caused even anguish to Kepler himself since it was common knowledge that we do not see things this way. Nevertheless, he stuck with his conclusion since – as he stated - geometry dictated this to be true and *"geometry could not be wrong"*. And, of course, as we know today he was right. But he also faced another problem of how we see near and far (not knowing that the lens could change in thickness). He posited that the distance between the lens and the retina had to change if a person would focus on a near or far object (others speculated that the cornea would change thickness or that the eye would elongate or shorten). This (and the other theories) turned out to be wrong. However, Kepler's theoretical considerations about the retinal image were proven to be correct by the German Jesuit priest and natural philosopher Christoph Scheiner (around 1600). He took a large animal eye and removed a small portion from its back and saw what Kepler had predicted. Viewing a candle he saw it upside down through this preparation. A schematic drawing of this preparation as pictured in a book (1637) by Descartes is shown below:

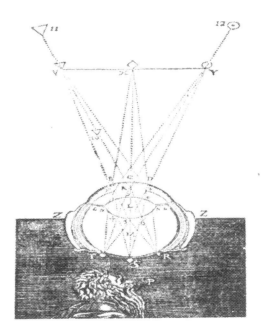

Figure 34

Scheiner and Descartes also suggested that the lens would change its thickness during accommodation from near to far and vice versa. This was finally proven experimentally to be correct by the English scholar Thomas Young (around 1800). Now the optics of the eye had been solved in that the cornea and the lens served as optical devices to project the picture accurately onto the retina (although still upside down and side reversed).

Up to this time, little progress had been made in understanding how we actually see. The importance of colors had been mentioned by ancient scholars but how we would see them was still a mystery. Interestingly, it has been claimed that the words for colors seem to appear quite late in the development of any language indicating that they did not play an important role in every day life. The ancient Greek scholars developed the two vision theories but had a different view of colors and might not even had a word for certain colors. The word for blue was kyanos or "cyan" but the ancient saga about the Trojan War described Hector's hair as cyan which most likely was not blue but dark. Honey or blood was called green or chloros and green probably meant fresh and moist (fresh wood is still described as green wood). Plato (about 400 BCE) said: "... *the several colors are formed, even if a man knew he would be foolish in telling, for he could not give any necessary reason, nor indeed any tolerable or probable explanation of them*". Later on, Greek scholars proposed that the basic colors were white, black, red and yellow and the other colors to be mixtures of the first. Aristotle made light shine through separate yellow and blue glass fragments and observed yellow and blue. Then he let the light shine through both fragments together and saw green. He concluded that a mixture of yellow and blue light resulted in green. Unfortunately, this was not correct because each time a light passes through a colored glass one of its spectral colors is removed. He then postulated three principal colors: red, green and violet (perhaps meaning blue), and the rest being mixtures of the three (which is surprisingly close to what we know today).

In the early medieval times in the western world, colors were a gift of the Lord and were interpreted to show his omnipresent. While colors were used extensively by artists, scholars did not concern themselves with their nature or how we would see them. This changed with Newton's discovery (see above) that light consisted of different colors (or better different wavelengths perceived as different colors). It was, however, still unknown how we see these different colors. Around 1780, the English scholar George Palmer posited that color vision is caused by light interacting with *"special particles"* in the retina to cause our color sensations (but he was also a clever inventor in that he constructed a lamp with a bluish glass ball around the yellow oil flame to obtain more true "day light' which was quickly used by tailors who could now see the "day light" colors of their works even at night). This was further extended by the English physician and scholar Thomas Young who did not think that the retina had *"special particles"* for every color but that there might only be three *"special particles"* and the German physician and scholar Hermann von Helmholtz around 1850 championed this same idea but proposed 5 *"special particles"*. Further experiments proofed Young to be correct and the three-chromatic color theory (blue, red and green) was now firmly established.

The English scientist John Dalton who lived around 1800 was color blind. He wrote: *"That part of the image which others call red appears to me little more than a shade or defect of light. After that the orange, yellow and green seem one colour which descends pretty uniformly from an intense to a rare yellow, making what I should call different shades of yellow"*. He postulated that the defect in color perception was caused by his ocular fluid to be bluish and therefore filtering out all the colors. He had his eyes examined after his death - but no blue fluid was detected.

It was not until 1875 that German scientists discovered while working on the isolated retina of excised frog eyes that their preparations changed colors during different light conditions or they would show a different color if looked at it by candle light (the only light source after sunset at this time) versus bright sun light. Exploring this color change, it was found to be produced by a special photosensitive chemical or pigment present in the photosensitive cells of the retina (rods, cones) which was then called rhodopsin. It then took until 1930 when scientists discovered that this rhodopsin consisted actually of two parts: a protein called opsin and a yellow organic chemical called a "chromophore" identified later as retinal which the human body makes from vitamin A. This explained the known fact that individuals with a vitamin A deficient diet and suffering from a vitamin A avitaminosis have trouble seeing. They also found that rhodopsin would split into the protein and the chromophore when exposed to light and would regenerate or combine again during darkness. Today, this process has been further expanded and a multitude of finely tuned biochemical reactions have been identified which occur in these cells. Electrophysiological studies during the middle and end of the 20th century measuring the response of individual photosensitive cells to various light waves confirmed that there were indeed three different kinds of cones each of them responding maximally to one particular wavelength of red, blue and green. This would result in the perception of these three colors. It was also found that excitation of more than one cone by other wave lengths caused the other colors to be seen.

But how these chemical changes in the photosensitive cells would transmit their information to the adjacent nerve cells still remained a mystery for quite a while. This process was discovered relatively late at the very end of the 20th century when researchers observed that certain chemicals would be released from light activated photosensitive cells which would keep adjacent nerve cells quiet but would trigger a nerve impulse if they would cease to be released. These nerve impulses would then be transmitted via the optic nerve into the brain. Thus, the last puzzle of the conversion of chemical reactions into electrical nerve impulses was solved and at present the finer details of this process are being worked out.

The deciphering of the visual processes of the brain was somewhat slower and it is still only incompletely understood even today. The involvement of the brain in seeing was recognized actually quite early on and the English scholar Fludd around 1600, for instance, speculated about a possible connection between the eyes and brain by presenting the picture (Figure 35) shown on the next page where seeing objects would give rise to our images and visual memories in the brain.

But how this worked remained unknown for quite some time. But physicians and scholars looked at individual brain structures now more carefully and tried to associate some of them with certain activities which in our case were the visual processes. In 1824, a French physician noticed that loss of vision occurred after damage to certain areas of the cortex suggesting that these parts might be the sites of sight. Around 1900, the American scientist Flexner showed that the visual neuronal

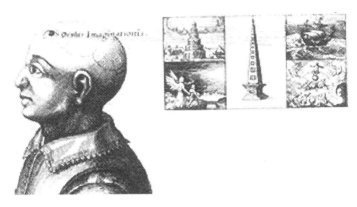

Figure 35

pathway from the eyes would lead to the lateral geniculate nucleus and from there to the striated area in the cortex. Around 1970, Hubel and Wiesel showed how these areas in the cortex responded to input from the excited retina. Using anesthetized animals and extremely fine electrodes inserted into specific areas of their brains, they could show the existence of certain "columns" and "layers" of neurons in their cortices which were involved in vision. By depriving small kittens of the use of one eye it was found that these areas in the brain corresponding to this eye would not develop properly (which is of major importance in understanding the human problem of amblyopia where the brain favors one eye over the other resulting in loss of stimulation of the brain area connected with the unused eye and underdevelopment or even loss of neuronal tissue). From there on a great deal of attention has been focused on these columns and layers and today we know that there are six layers containing billions of nerve cells which form small networks which are then integrated into larger networks. Simultaneously, clinical studies of patients who had brain trauma or strokes in these areas showed that some patients would suffer from visual agnosia which includes the inability to identify, draw or copy common objects. It was first thought (around 1990) that this was the result of bad eye sight. Later on, the problem was placed into certain areas of the brain. This finally led to the recognition and identification of special visual areas in the human cortex which are in steady communication and which make it finally possible to correctly see, identify, describe and remember people, animals or objects.

Over the last few years, we have learned a lot about our visual processes. We understand the optics of the eye very well and we have pretty much deciphered how the waves are converted into chemical reactions and then into electrical activity in the retina. However, we are just at the beginning of understanding the visual processes of the brain. These last processes are still a mystery- how does electrical activity produce a meaningful visual image in our brain and how is it possible that we see it then outside our brain?

Medicine and Ocular Medicine. From the beginning of history, people must have suffered from a variety of health problems caused by accidents, tribal warfare and diseases including problems with their eyes such as impaired vision or blindness. Since no records are available from prehistoric times, such problems can only be surmised from skeletons found in various places. Since the eyes had disappeared from the skulls nothing is known about ocular diseases from these times.

Early records from the ancient civilizations like those of the Babylonians, Indians, Chinese, Egyptians, Greeks and Romans verified the existence of a fair number of health problems including those afflicting the eyes. It is known that these ancient people suffered from a wide variety of eye problems and diseases but since often only ocular symptoms were described or names of diseases were given which cannot be translated into our medical terms of today it is uncertain which specific diseases had been present and were prevalent. Nevertheless, our ancient ancestors tried to find causes as well as cures for these ailments. In the beginning, the causes of illnesses and problems of the body and eye were mostly of supernatural origin. For instance, a good god was neglected or offended by an individual and the punishment was sickness of the body and the eye. In addition, bad gods and demons could also cause sickness and eye problems just to torment and torture people. The old Sumerians had over 1000 demons that could harm people in various ways. The ancient Chinese felt that neglected ancestors could cause body and eye problems. Thus, the help of priests and priestesses or other religious individuals had to be sought and the remedy and cure would be to ask the offended gods for forgiveness or to beg good gods for help to remove the curse of bad gods or demons through prayers, atonement, sacrifices and rituals. The old Greeks had special temples where sick people could regain health through a "temple sleep'. Stories were then published and distributed among the population where a patient was miraculous cured through this therapy but then became sick again when he refused to give a monetary reward to the temple (indicating a hidden threat not to skip payment). Even today certain religious groups feel that diseases are God's punishment for sins and the remedy consists of prayers with medications to be thought as secondary remedies or even worthless and are shunned.

These rituals were sometimes helped by consulting worldly healers and physicians. They would use herbs, minerals, animal and human body parts, wine, mother's milk, urine and other "medications" which in most cases might have done more harm than good. Nevertheless, ancient Greek physicians like Hippocrates (he supposedly lived around 400 BCE but his teachings were not written down and compiled until centuries later and are most likely his as well as those of other physicians) stressed a good diet, exercise and sufficient sleep which we still emphasize today as good preventive measures as well as helping in curing a disease. Greek physicians like Hippocrates also proposed that health was the result of a balance of four natural humors in the body, namely black and yellow bile, phlegm and blood and any imbalance of them would cause certain illnesses in the body and the eye. Thus, treatment intended to restore the original balance by reducing the excess of one humor (e.g. excess blood was reduced by blood letting or phlebotomy) or by strengthening of a weakened humor (e.g. with certain foods, sleep, exercise and medications).

Ancient Egyptians suffered from many eye diseases one of which was trachoma (an infectious eye disease) and old records talked about Egypt as the "land of blindness". Causes and treatments were mostly mystical and religious. An ancient text describes the following "treatment" of an eye problem: *"Welcome, this eye of Horus, the magnificent, which is in the eye of Horus, which is created, to abolish the influence of a god, the influence of a goddess, a male opponent, a female opponent, a male dead, a female dead, a male enemy, a female enemy which affected adversely both eyes of the man who is under my fingers. Protection, protection, protection"*. Prayers, rituals and mostly worthless – sometimes even dangerous - medications were used. A remedy for a lid hair which had curled from the lid into and caused irritation and damage to the eye was treated by the old Egyptians as follows: *"Another* [remedy] *to drive out curling up the hair in the eye: incense blood of lizard 1, blood of bat 1. Pull out the hair. Apply to it so it gets well"*.

Ancient physicians in India way before the birth of Christ had already developed a cure for cataracts. They would introduce a needle into the eye and push down to restore sight (as we know today to remove the clouded lens from the path of light). This was sometimes successful although a lot of eyes got lost or became blind due to infections. However, since this procedure was usually only performed if the eye had already become blind, even a modest cure rate was already a success. Interestingly, this method of "couching" the cataract was the standard method used in most countries including Europe and later on America for the next 2000 years and was still practiced in rural areas of India until recently.

Ancient Chinese physicians invented acupuncture and used this technique since about 800 BCE (acupuncture needles were discovered dating back to this time). Interestingly, acupuncture is still being performed in many countries today albeit little for ocular problems. They also invented moxibustion where a small amount of an herb is burned on the skin of the patient causing a blister which was believed to restore health. This procedure again was used well into the late medieval ages. They also believed that diseases of the eye were the extensions of bodily diseases.

Roman physicians like Galen (about 150 CE) and Celsus (about 100 CE) summarized Greek thinking in a number of medical texts and added some of their own observations as well. These writings became the standard texts in the western world for the next 1500 years. Diseases including those of the eye were still thought to be caused by an imbalance of the four humors which continued to be the basis of all pathological processes. They described a large number of ocular diseases; unfortunately their cures were mostly ineffective or even dangerous. Interestingly Galen already mentions:*" so that when our eye looks at the inflamed eye of a patient we catch the inflammation ourselves"* recognizing the infectious nature of many ocular diseases.

The rise of Christianity in the western world during the medieval ages (about 400-1400) promoted again divine causes of diseases which were now viewed once more as godly punishment for a sinful life. Each of the deadly sins caused a specific illness. Sometimes diseases and epidemics were blamed on heathens, Jews and atheists. In the early and middle medieval ages, the Church taught that the body belonged to God and only God could keep such a body healthy, inflict a disease or remove a disease from the body. Physicians were only the servants of God needing divine help to cure the patient. Thus, medical treatment always involved prayers. Church doctrine was to save the soul first and the body later and only then if it did not hurt the soul. However, Christian religion dictated taking care of people and the monasteries were often hospitals as well: "*Before all things and above all things, care must be taken of the sick, so that they will be served as if they were Christ in person; for He Himself said, "I was sick, and you visited me".* St. Augustine stated around 400 that medical treatment is useful and beneficial, but diseases are God-given exhortations and needed mostly religious treatment: "*As sickness of the body may sometimes be the result of sin ... since the soul is much more precious than the body, we forbid any physician, under pain of anathema, to prescribe anything for the bodily health of a sick person that may endanger his soul.".* Thus, prayers and the help of the Church were sought first as cures as was self-punishment. During the times of the Plague, people would punish themselves to end the epidemic – well known were the flagellants who would whip their backs bloody with ropes and branches.

Physicians would treat eye diseases with phlebotomy and cauterizing the temples to prevent the "*flow of bad humors from the brain into the eye*". They would use many medications which were often concocted secretly and were mostly worthless. They consisted of minerals, herbs, animal body parts, as well as human fluids like urine or mother's milk. In the later medieval ages, Egyptian mummy parts were used since they were believed to have miraculous healing powers. Since the demand soon outstripped the supply, unscrupulous merchants often substituted the dried flesh from executed criminals. An example of the medical treatment of an eye problem was: "*A good method is: take a shed snake skin, ground with a silver – or saliva – leaf introduced into fistula twice daily and a sage leaf bound to either foot. In the name of the Father say: as Christ descended from heaven into the uterus of a virgin, may this fistula descend from the eye to the foot. Say it three times*". Another recipe read as follows: *"For preserving and improving vision in age and other conditions, take a little skimmed honey. Place it in a glass flask and mix it with bile of rabbit and chicken and other birds that make a living by hunting. Leave it in the sun for nine days and nights. Let it be diluted by dew. Finally, place it in the eyes"*. However, the success of medications was always dependent on God's will – only if God wanted the medication to work would it work (which left the physician and medication of the hook since failure was only caused by God who did not want the medication to work). Many sandstone statues of saints from these times lack their eyes because people removed them and mixed the ground sandstone eyes into ointments for ocular applications. Medications were often applied in – what to us seems a strange way – to objects. A special "wound salve" was used – but not on the body but on the part of the object which had caused the wound. It consisted of ground-up earthworms, iron oxide, pig's brain and powdered mummy parts. In addition, amulets were used frequently to prevent or to cure diseases and illnesses (while this might sound bizarre, a look at the internet will tell you that you still can buy many amulets today which are claimed to prevent or even cure certain illnesses). Astrology played a major and significant role in surgical and medical treatments. Physicians would rely on the constellation of the stars and planets since they were controlled by God and the Lord would send through their constellation certain signals to the physician in how to prevent or to cure a disease. Again, it should not be forgotten that even today a fair number of people believe in the powers inherent in astrology.

While physicians would treat diseases of the eye, eye surgery was left to barber/surgeons called oculists. Oculists would obtain their training by another oculist or would just proclaim themselves as an oculist. They would mostly remove cataracts by "couching" (or depressing the cataract with a needle inserted into the affected eye) but would also treat eye diseases with "drugs". This was often performed at market fairs. They would often do the cataract surgery and then recommend bed rest for a few days with the eyes tightly bandaged – during which time they quickly skipped the village or town. These oculists often led a dangerous life as it has been recorded that the Bohemian King John of Luxemburg was infected with trachoma (a special eye infection) in

1337. A French oculist who could not help him was tied up in a sack and thrown into the river Odra.

However, something very important and indeed beneficial happened during this time which still is in existence today. This was the advent of spectacles. Around 1000, people started to use "reading stones" (magnifying lenses) which would help older individuals with vision problems. Around 1300, the art of grinding lenses had improved and the first spectacles appeared in Italy at this time (roidi da ogli or slabs for the eyes). They were used at first by the educated for presbyopia but soon spectacles for correcting myopia followed. The use of spectacles spread rapidly since now more people started to read (see next page). Their designs changed and were constantly improved. Lenses were mounted at first in leather, wood, bone or even light steel. The rich preferred hand-held spectacles with frames of gold and silver and adorned with precious stones. Designs with a rigid nose bridge appeared about 1600 followed by rigid extensions to the ears and Benjamin Franklin invented in the USA the first bifocals by cementing two lenses together.

In contrast, medicine and ocular medicine flourished in the Islamic nation during these times and Baghdad became the center of science and medicine. While the humeral theory of medicine was still accepted, scholars stressed the importance of anatomy for the understanding of the human body (which was sadly neglected in the western world because the Church basically prohibited dissections). Many hospitals were established throughout the Islamic country since Islam dictated donations from the wealthy for the treatment of the sick. These hospitals were foremost centers for medical treatment and education (while this was only a minor function in the monasteries in the western world). Interestingly, not only Islamic but also Christian and Jewish physicians were working in these hospitals. As mentioned earlier, the importance of Islamic medicine declined after 1000 as religious thoughts became dominant and took preference in science and medicine.

A major change occurred in the Western world around 1500 with the beginning of the Renaissance. Sciences and medicine started to be reawakened and to slowly free themselves from the shackles of the ancient thinking and traditions. In addition, the influence of the Church on medicine and science began to wane. Observations, experimentations and observations started to replace many of the old scientific and medical beliefs which were now proven to be outdated and wrong. The Swiss/German physician Paracelsus (1493/1494 to 1541) broke with traditional medicine and superstition and introduced "iatrochemistry" into medicine replacing the four humors with chemical reactions in the body which went wrong during diseases (for instance, he wrote that the miner's lung disease was not caused by demons in the mountains offended by the drilling into their home but by the dust the miners inhaled during their labor).

During this time two major events occurred which had an enormous impact on medicine (as well as science in general). In 1450, Johannes Gutenberg invented the printing press based on movable letters. This offered the possibility of printing books rapidly (the old presses were cumbersome and allowed the printing of only a few copies) and faultlessly (hand written copies often contained copying errors). Now medical and scientific (as well as other) information could be printed accurately and distributed quickly among a large readership. An additional benefit was that the printing industry encouraged more education for the ordinary public because only people who could read would buy their books. Medical knowledge restricted to a few physicians until then could now be distributed rapidly and read by many in different countries. The second event was the discovery of the Americas and other parts of the world until then unknown territories. The discoverers brought with them news about other cultures (including medicine) as well as many new plants and herbs some of which had indeed healing powers (like quinine which had fever reducing properties and coca leaves from which later on cocaine was isolated and used as a local anesthetic).

The first real breakthrough for ocular medicine occurred in 1583 when the German oculist Georg Bartisch published his textbook on ocular diseases and their treatments in a book called "Augendienst" (Eye Service) written in German (a break with the old tradition of writing books in Latin). Many scholars consider this book the first Textbook of Ophthalmology. He had learned his trade from other oculists as an apprentice and after "graduating" worked as an oculist. He traveled through the country performing his various eye operations on market fairs and - based on his success and reputation - was later on named royal oculist and stone cutter to the King of Saxony (stone cutter referred to removal of bladder stones which oculists also did by sticking a knife just above the anus into the bladder and then removing the stones with their fingers). He described some of the eye operations performed at this time quite in detail, gave a list of medications for various ocular ailments and added some new procedures which he had invented. The first picture (Figure 36) shows preparation for major ocular surgery by tying down the patient (because anesthetics were not known at this time except alcohol and morphine which are not very effective in reducing pain during surgery). Cataract operations would still be done according to the ancient Indian procedure of "couching" in that a needle would be stuck sideways into the eye and then pushed down. This operation would only be performed if the eye was completely blind so the few people who experienced a successful operation and could see again felt it was worth the surgery while the rest had nothing to lose. A good cataract "sticker" could do this procedure within a minute or less. This practice of 'couching" was the only cataract operation done at the time – with the drawbacks that the lens might move up again later on and the operation had to be repeated and that many eyes were lost due to infections and inflammations.

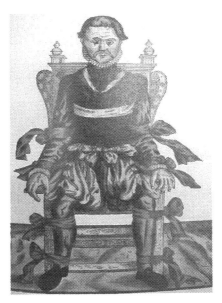

Figure 36

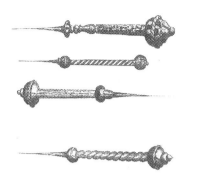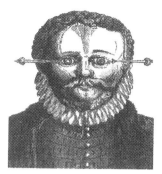

Figure 37

The picture above (Figure 37) shows the needles on the left and the procedure on the right. This procedure was refined later on in order to prevent the re-emergence of the lens in that the lens was removed with tweezers through a cut in the eye. Although being more successful, it took a longer time and caused more pain and, thus, was only slowly accepted by oculists and physicians as well as patients. It finally became the procedure of choice after general anesthetics like chloroform and ether had been discovered and cocaine was found to be an excellent local anesthetic in the eye in 1880. These drugs preventing pain and discomfort allowed now the surgeon to substitute speed for accuracy. Thus, general and local anesthetics opened up a new approach in surgery and helped greatly in the development of improved general and ocular surgical procedures. They also required now barber/surgeons who were usually not physicians up to this time and needed little knowledge of anatomy – since speed was the only requirement of a good surgeon – to become more educated anatomically and medically which helped them later to become accepted by physicians forming eventually an alliance.

Until 1850, glaucoma was untreatable and would lead eventually to blindness. Ophthalmologists and oculist knew at this time already that a 'blind" eye caused by glaucoma could not be "couched" successfully and would not treat such patients. At this time, the German physician von Graefe discovered that excision of a piece of the iris (iridectomy) could be used to treat glaucoma effectively. Unfortunately, this procedure was only slowly adapted by ophthalmologists with the result that many eyes got lost which could have been saved. After 1875, the first somewhat effective drugs to treat this problem were discovered and used.

The middle of the 19th century proved to be again a turning point in medicine including ophthalmology. At this time, scientific and medical progress started to accelerate at a faster and faster pace with new discoveries and improved medical treatments appearing almost yearly. One of these was the invention of the ophthalmoscope by the German physician von Helmholtz around 1850 which allowed now physicians for the first time to see into the eye and to observe the posterior (background of the eye) structures of the eyes of their patients. Now diseases of the inner eye could be detected early and later on be treated before significant damage had occurred. But there were very few effective medications except atropine to dilate the pupil and pilocarpine to treat open angle glaucoma.

Education and practice of physicians was re-examined at this time and major changes were instituted. Physicians in America up to 1900 were educated at universities with vastly varying standards but also could receive their education by serving an apprenticeship with an established physician. After 1900, a university education for physicians was required and medical schools had to adhere to certain standards. Students soon had to pass nationwide tests and physicians are now required to pass examinations to become board certified and have to constantly update their knowledge during their practice.

Unfortunately, drugs were still poorly controlled at this time until some major catastrophes occurred. In the USA in 1937, the drug sulfonamide was manufactured and distributed in a liquid form using diethylene glycol as solvent which had not been tested for toxicity before and turned out to be highly toxic. This preparation killed 107 adults and children. In1955, 260 people contracted polio after receiving a polio vaccine where the virus had not been properly inactivated. This prompted the establishment of the Food and Drug Administration or FDA as a controlling agency under the auspices of the National Institutes of Health. This agency now controls the introduction of new drugs and their manufacturing and distribution only after the manufacturer had convinced a panel of experts that the drug is indeed efficacious and relatively safe or it is made evident that its benefits clearly outweigh its risks. Every prescription drug on the market is then constantly surveyed and if health problems arise the FDA tells the manufacturers to withdraw the drug from the market. Unfortunately, this is not required of alternative medications which are not controlled as to efficacy and toxicity. They are mostly ineffective but also can be dangerous. Prescription drug use is being aided by better educated pharmacists who can survey the medications a patient takes, can spot dangerous drug or food interactions and can advise the patient on the right use of their prescribed medications. Nurses and medical technicians are now highly trained and experienced professionals. A number of highly effective technical procedures like CAT and MRI scans are available to detect early health problems which can often be corrected before irreparable damage occurs.

During the last 50 years – well within the lives of many of us – major advances occurred in ocular medicine and the restoration of vision. Contact lenses started to replace spectacles. Contact lenses had been experimented with already in the late 19th century but the first usable contact lens was born in 1948 and the hard plastic lenses were introduced in the 1970s. The extended wear lenses and the gas permeable lenses made their appearance in the 1980s. During this time implantable lenses after cataract surgery were developed and quite recently multi focal lenses can be implanted which do not require the use of eye glasses. Vision correction by reshaping of the cornea started in the 1970s with making cuts into the cornea which would then change its curvature and restore better refraction. This was soon followed by Lasik and Lasek surgery in the 1980s which was made possible by advanced laser technologies. These procedures are now used safely and successfully. Cataract operations which in the 1970s required hospitalization with sandbags around the head for several days became an outpatient procedure with the cataract extraction done within a few minutes. Corneal transplantations became a routine procedure and they are restoring the vision in many patients (such a procedure had been tried for the first time in 1905 by the Austrian physician Zirm who successfully transplanted the cornea of a young boy who accidentally had died into the eye of a laborer who had lost his cornea due to chemical exposure).Similarly, retinal detachment has lost its dire consequence of severe vision impairment or blindness due to the development of various procedure to re-attach a torn and loose retina. Bacterial eye infections for which there was no effective treatment until 1935 when the first sulfa drug and 1945 when penicillin were introduced are now being treated with quite a large number of effective medications. Viral infections could not be treated until around 1960 when the first two antiviral drugs were introduced soon to be followed by a large number of similar drugs. Similarly, the first antifungal drugs were introduced at this time. Up to 1945, cancers were treated by surgery or removal of the eye. After this time the first anticancer drugs were introduced (after pharmacologists investigating certain toxic warfare agents noted that they would not only kill the animals but would also depress their lymph nodes and bone marrow – some were later tried successfully in lymphomas) and again the bulk of the newer and more effective agents were introduced after 1970 to treat cancers of the body and eye. The first effective and least toxic antiglaucoma drug –timolol – was not introduced until around 1980 and again the bulk of the newer drugs used today to treat glaucoma was discovered and used only after 1990 (although pilocarpine in the treatment of glaucoma had been used around 1900 but this drug is not tolerated well by many patients). Macular degeneration which affects a large number of older people and which caused often early vision impairment or blindness can now be partially treated. In particular, drugs have become available since 2000 which can significantly slow the progression of this disorder, prevent its major complications and extent normal vision for years. Looking at ocular medicine today, it can be said that we have come a long, long way and are finally at a stage where we can successfully prevent and/or treat many ocular problems which only fifty years ago would have been untreatable or where only treatable with considerable risk to the patient.

It is interesting to recognize that the major advances made in ocular medicine as we enjoy them today were mostly achieved within the last 50-100 years of a period of about 4500 years of recorded human history. About 95% of today's successful eye treatments and operations were developed within the last 2.5 % of recorded human history. For about 3900 years, humans suffered from many eye ailments, diseases and problems some of which caused considerable discomfort and great pain while others led to blindness. Most of these can now be prevented, cured or reduced in severity and the vision of many eyes can be saved. We are indeed lucky to live today!

The Vision of Animals

Vision is a major part of human sensation with the other senses like hearing, smell, touch and taste only serving moderate to minor roles. Animals also use vision with some being inferior and other being superior to humans. However, vision is often not their primary and dominant sense. Many animals use smell as their major sense and some have developed "senses" which humans do not posses. The following paragraphs describe the visual system of various animal species showing how each individual species has developed a particular and different visual system which is most advantageous and beneficial for its survival and reproduction.

In order to examine vision in the animal kingdom, the eye is easily dissected and its various structures and their specific functions can be relatively easily identified. Based on our knowledge of the human eye interferences can then easily be made and are relatively accurate. This is a bit more difficult with an animal brain where we can look at the anatomy and measure its size and dissect its matter but are still relatively unsure about the specific functions of such individual structures except perhaps in some laboratory animals – like rats, cats or monkeys - which have been scientifically studied and which have given us a lot of information in how the human brain works. We must assume that the central visual processes in the various wild species work similar to those of the laboratory animals and the human brain.

Animals which live in caves or in other dark areas where vision is not necessary are often completely blind such as the blind Texas salamander, blind flatworms, eyeless shrimp, eyeless fish, cave beetles or cave crayfish. Some species of cave fish are born with eyes but then skin just grows over them and the eyes degenerate completely because there is no need for sight in the pitch-black world of their environment. Instead they did develop extremely sensitive back fins which allow them to navigate accurately with the help of water currents. However, it was recently discovered when these fish were mated with seeing fish from a different environment, their first generation off-springs would keep the eyes and would preserve their vision. In another experiment lenses from seeing fish were implanted into blind fish and were found to develop into eyes. They could most likely not see with these eyes but it shows that they still have the inherent genetic ability to form eyes but just do not do so since they are useless in their dark environment.

Worms have no eyes but have light sensitive cells on their body. If an earthworm has been in the dark and is then exposed to sun light, it will quickly try to move away from the light back into darkness. A night crawler will immediately retract into its burrow if you shine a flashlight on it. This movement is called phototaxis and is probably the most primitive from of vision distinguishing only between light and dark.

Some insects like termites and some ants are almost or completely blind and yet function astonishingly well. Other insects have developed very interesting eyes called compound eyes. A compound eye consists of thousands of tiny independent photoreception units – called ommatidia. They are typically hexagonal in cross section, approximately ten times longer than wide and the outer part is larger than the inner part. At the outer surface there is a cornea. Below is a pseudocone (precursor to a lens??) which acts to further focus the light. This is followed by special long thin cells which are the photosensitive cells. They react only to that part of the environment directly in front of them. From there, nerve cells project to the brain. Such a compound eye with its multitude of ommatidia is shown below:

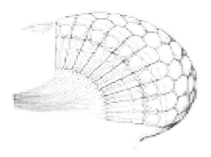

Figure 38

The image processed by the brain is then a combination of the inputs of these thousands of units. The image is either a composite or a single picture of the seen object. They have some color vision but usually a poor image resolution while, however, covering a large visual field. They can detect movements quickly – a fact known to us if you like to swat a fly which usually escapes the blow of our swatter because it can detect its movement way before it is being struck. Some spiders surpass us by having eight eyes. Some spiders synthesize a light sensitive membrane in their eyes during the night to see better in dim light and destroy this membrane during the day. Bees are somewhat of an exception among insects because bees have – similar to us – tri-colored vision. They are very good in seeing different colors and do this by using each of the 6,300 individual ommatidia of their compound eye. They also use vision as a way to communicate. We all know about the bee dance where an incoming bee to the hive communicates to its sisters where food can be found by performing a somewhat circular dance – this tells the other bees the direction, the distance and the quantity of available food. The firefly uses light and vision to find a mate. During courtship, the male flashes a sequence of lights produced by two specific chemicals (luciferin and luciferase) to be seen and answered – hopefully – by a female. Among the different species of fireflies each has its own sequence and rhythm (and some ancient people kept fireflies in their house at night as a source of light). It is interesting that some insects possess color vision which is not present or present only in an undeveloped way in lower mammals and seems to only appear more completely in higher primates. Recently, a fly was discovered which was trapped in amber hundred million years ago which had three eyes – apparently, evolution felt that two eyes were as efficient as three eyes and the genes for the third eye were eventually abandoned.

Among fish, vision also varies with some having better while others having poorer vision. Most fish cannot see more than a hundred meters. Important differences between the human and fish eye are the absence of lids and the shape of the cornea and the lens. The cornea does not need to be highly refractive because there is very little difference between the water on the outside and the watery fluid inside the eye (while in humans the outside is air). Similarly, the lens is also adjusted to the outside medium water (our lens does not work well in water – as we all know from swimming under water). Thus, the fish eye has adapted to this special environment. Because of its spherical shape the lens protrudes through the iris which in most fishes is also fixed or contracts very slowly. Some fish can move their lenses back and forth to accommodate. Some have even two lenses, one on the outside and one on the inside of the eye. The Schuetzenfisch which is a surface water fish has two retinas so that half the eye under water uses one and the other in the air uses the other retina so that these fish always can see simultaneously well in and above the water. The flounder has developed the "wandering eye " – a very young flounder swims like most fish with one eye on each side of the body but as it ages it will lay on one side on the ground of the ocean. Now one eye migrates to the other side so that two eyes are on the upper side to survey what is above. The size of the eyes also varies greatly among fish depending if they live closer to the surface or in darker water with the latter usually having bigger eyes to catch more of the few light rays present. Some fish are able to roll their eyes backward for a complete rear view – which humans cannot do. Fish also can have different rods. Some fish can move their rods physically to the front to increase their sensitivity. Fish have less sensitive cones and can see colors but not as distinct as humans (and colors disappear anyhow in deep water). Some fish can have special cones – fish with such cones can see infrared or ultraviolet light which we cannot see. Here, the gold fish has four different cones and can see, for instance, green objects in a changing ambient light. The mantis shrimp has ten different color receptors including infrared sensitive cones. Infrared vision improves their vision since the long infrared wave lengths are less scattered in water – as we know from a "red" sun set where all the other colors except red are scattered by clouds. The eye of the octopus has taken a different evolutionary route since this creature has the rods and cones almost exclusively in front of the nerve cells (while this is of course the opposite in all other eyes) . The octopus therefore has no blind spot because the nerve cells leave from behind the photosensitive cells. Recently, a rare fish was discovered with a transparent head. This fish could look ahead but could also look through its own skull up to spot food or predators. Recently, it was found that the eye of the deep-sea dragon fish can see red light because they contain chlorophyll (which is usually only found in plants) and which allows the fish to see red. As one descends deeper and deeper into the ocean, it becomes darker and darker until there is eternal night. However, it is not truly dark because organisms living at this depth can create their own light called bioluminescence. Bioluminescence is the production and emission of light by certain tissues using special chemical reactions (like the firefly). It is estimated that ninety percent of deep-sea marine life produces and uses this bioluminescence in one form or another. Thus, the darkness is interrupted with a multitude of blue, orange or green flashes. They are used to warn of danger, to find a mate or to secure food. Some fish glow at their bellies so that they can find food below but cannot be seen by predators swimming above. Such bioluminescent flashes are sometimes used to scare predators and enhance survival. If a jelly-fish is caught by a predator, it starts to glow in the hope that it will attract a bigger predator which will eat the smaller one and free the jelly-fish. Other creatures use special bioluminescence to find each other. Some fish can enhance this bioluminescence. The spook fish has "four" eyes – but it actually only has two eyes and the other two "eyes" are mirrors which direct the dim bioluminescence into the real eyes so that the fish can spot prey more easily. This secret world is now being explored by using spy cameras which sit on the ocean floor and record the bioluminescence from these creatures. These are beautiful examples of how living organisms adapt to their environments no matter how harsh and different they may be.

Reptiles have eyes similar to that of humans except that they possess a nictitating membrane which is a third membrane over the eye lubricating and protecting the eye in addition to the two other eye lids. Some lizards have multicolored oil droplets in their photoreceptors so that they can perceive some colors better. Many species are able to see higher or lower wavelengths than can humans. Some have the slit-like pupil which contracts into a very narrow vertical slit composed of a linear array of very small dots which enhances vision (like humans who are nearsighted will often squint in order to improve their vision). Many amphibians like the frog have bulging eyes which they close by retracting the eyeballs back into the socket (and the eye balls in the frog also help in swallowing since they push food down).

Marine mammals like sea lions must see both under water and on land where the medium is either water or air and light is refracted differently in these media. It has been suggested that these animals are more water adapted and compensate for this on land by closing their pupils to a small slit which increases their visual acuity. Some marine mammals have only one type of cones and hence have poor color vision.

The eyes of birds are more similar to that of humans but again show some differences. The eye of a bird is much larger compared to body size amounting to about 10 % in some birds (with only 1% for humans). A bird's eye is tightly fitted into its skull and it is only capable of very limited movements. Thus, birds have to move their heads for better views of their surroundings. Their eyes have also a nictitating membrane. In some birds the nictitating membrane is translucent so that the bird can see while the eye is covered. The iris and lens are similar to those of humans and – like humans – birds can vary the thickness of the lens. The eyes of predatory birds are in the front to provide good binocular vision to focus on the prey. Some have a special structure in the eye which we humans do not have. This structure extends from the retina to the lens and is rich in blood vessels. This supplies parts of the eye with oxygen and nutrients so that the retina needs less blood vessels resulting in less light scattering and sharper vision. Non-predatory birds have the eyes on the side so that they have excellent field vision covering up to and in some cases exceeding 360 degrees to spot approaching predators. These birds watch you with one eye while the other eye screens the opposing side. In some birds such as hawks, kingfishers and swallows, the eye has two foveas, one for viewing sideways and one for viewing forward. Some raptors or birds of prey have many more rods in the fovea – a human has about 200 000 light sensitive cells per square millimeter while eagles might have 1 000 000. This gives these birds a distance vision at least five times better than ours and these birds flying at a height of 1000 feet can cover an area of almost three square miles and still can spot their prey. Birds can have up to five different types of cones (we only have three) which allows them to see certain colors and their individuals shades better than we can. Some cones of these birds allow them to see ultraviolet light – which we cannot perceive. In addition, the eyes of certain sea birds contain droplets of red oil in their eyes to cut out the blue light which scatters up from the sea and can disturb their vision. This makes it easier for them to discern small objects and prey floating on or flying near the ocean or water surface.

Mammals have an eye which again is quite similar to the human eye. One of the main difference is that the lens is usually much less flexible than that of the human eye and that in large animals the fovea which is about one square mm in humans can expand to a band which is much larger and can reach and extend to fifty square mm. The position of the two eyes will again vary depending if the animal is a predator or prey. Predators have their eyes in front. They can focus excellently in front to catch prey but have a wide blind area around and behind which can be tolerated since they have no or few predators. Grazing animals which are mostly prey have their eyes on the side. Their blind spots are small and just in front of the nose and in the back allowing them a much wider area of vision and, thus, they can spot predators more readily which often approach from behind or from the side.

Interestingly, the rabbit has no blind spot in the back and all around vision. These animals have double mono vision or the brain receives and sees two pictures – one with the left and one with the right eye (the human brain fuses both pictures from each eye together into one picture). Tigers and our house cats possess many more rods but fewer cones indicating sharper acuity but less color vision. They see objects more gray with some shades of colors. At the back of their eyes they have a mirror-like membrane called a tapetum (this is why cats' eyes glow when hit by light in the dark). It reflects the light passing through the rods back to the rods a second time, this time in the opposite direction. The combination of the elliptical pupils and the tapetum permit cats to see extremely well in near darkness. It is estimated that at night they see six times better than humans. Similar, dogs have more rods and again fewer cones. However, their color vision seems to be better than that of cats although most of their objects are seen as gray with some color shades. However, animals often focus differently on near and distant objects. The horse, for instance, is not able to focus by changing the thickness of the lens as much as we do. It moves its head up and down until the object comes into focus on its retina. If it lowers the head and gazes through the upper portion of the eye, it can focus on distant objects. It will raise its head and look through the lower portion of the eye when it will look at something close. With the eye in the midway position both distant and close objects can be in focus at the same time. Giraffes have very keen vision and it has been estimated they can spot a mate at a distance of over one half mile. Monkeys do have color vision which varies among species with the orangutan being thought to come closest to humans. Some animals are born with almost fully functioning eyes and brains and can use both very quickly which might be necessary for their survival. A gazelle born in the wild must be able to see and run quickly to escape ever present predators. In contrast some animals are born blind and their eyes and brains develop only slowly. This is probably so that they do not wander away while the parents forage for food.

Sometimes "eyes" are not used for seeing but for other purposes. They can be used for protection. Some butterflies have two big "eye" markings on its wings. They seem to warn and repel predators since experiments have shown that butterflies whose "eyes" were painted over were much more frequently eaten as compared to butterflies with exposed "eyes":

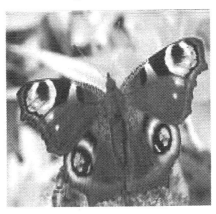

Figure 39

Colors can also fool predators in that certain creatures show colors very close to the colors of their environments and, in some case, will change colors like frogs or chameleons to always be in agreement with the colors of their environment and to remain undetected. Non-venomous snakes have evolved with colored skins which closely resemble those of venomous snakes and hope to warn predators to stay away. Some fish use their eyes as a warning to repel other male fish from their territory. These fish roll their eyes back until a reflecting part is exposed which reflects UV light (eyes start to glow) as a warning signal for the intruder. Light is used to feed like in the case of the anglerfish which has a glowing tissue hanging out of its mouth to attract prey.

Following the optics and physiology of the eye, the next step would be an examination of the central processing part of vision or the brain. Almost all living organisms possess single nerve cells, small and larger clusters of such nerve cells or finally brains which vary from being tiny as in insects to that of elephants which can weigh up to five kg (although based on body size it is still "smaller" than the human brain). Brains among higher animals look alike although they vary in size, weight and distribution of individual brain areas. From a visual point of view, visual brain areas of higher animals – we know little about insects and lower animals – are qualitatively similar to those of humans although they do differ in size. There are exceptions. The optic nerves in the brains of birds do not cross partially but the left nerve goes exclusively to the left and the right nerve to the right side of the brain.

While the animal (and human) brain looks like an organ with mirror symmetry it actually shows a strong internal lateralization for certain activities as we know from humans. Even bees have their preferences. Bees with their left eyes covered with a tiny patch and only using their right eyes learned quickly to find a new food source while bees with their right eyes covered and only using their left eyes had considerable trouble to do so. Toads have been found to "see" insects better on the right side while often ignoring those on the left side. However, they seem to avoid predators easier if they approach from the left. Birds have been shown to use their left side to find food and the right side to spot predators. Parrots have been observed to pick up things with the left foot but go after prey with the right one. Zebra fish seem to look at new objects with their right eye and at familiar things with the left one. Higher animals show similar characteristics in that monkeys prefer mostly the right hand while observing and performing certain visual tasks. However, how these animals interpret what they see is much more difficult to asses and often is based on assumptions and speculations. Apparently, left-right side preferences are an evolutionary matter which we inherited from our ancestors – the insects and animals.

It is astonishing how all the complex behavior of an ant (see later) or a bee is accomplished by a brain which can hardly be seen by the naked eye. These brain cells in the bee can interpret the special movements or "dance" of their sister telling them not only the location and but also the quantity of a food source. This tiny brain can distinguish up to 300 separate flashes of light per second – which we can not do – and use this information during their flight to and from food sources. It has even been claimed that bees recognize faces – bees learned to associate a certain face with a sugar solution and another face with water and followed the face which was attached to the sugar solution.

As one moves up the ladder, reptiles and fish have many more neurons in their brains which fulfill the basic but necessary functions for their bearers. These more primitive brains are sometimes referred to as "old brains" (since they originated first during evolution). The brain of a 200 kg alligator weighs about 14 g (compared with the 30 g brain of a four kg heavy cat). Reptiles and some fish do not have many visual capabilities and often rely on sight location or movement without a solid interpretation of what is moving. They will catch something and the taste then might or might not tell them if it is eatable. This is why upon opening of a dead alligator or shark one will find in the stomach eatable and uneatable pieces and objects mixed together. It has been said that a frog in a jar surrounded by dead flies would starve to death because it can only see moving flies. Experiments have shown that the brains of toads can even recognize and memorize movement correlations. They seem to recognize movements from the side as dangerous – since predators prefer this side for an attack - and frontal movements as beneficial – since a prey moves usually away in front of the toad.

These primitive brain areas are still present and function in higher animals and humans. Animals will spot moving prey or predators much more readily than quiet ones. Newborn gazelles when left alone will lie very quiet to avoid being detected by a predator. Documentary films have shown that a lion when discovering such a gazelle will not kill it until it starts to move. These animal brains respond much quicker to environmental challenges than do human brains. This is an important asset in catching prey or surviving the constant threat of predators. Such an animal brain might see and comprehend something at one glance whereas humans might need a couple of glances. Nevertheless, we humans also have inherited this capability because we might not see a bird in the tree unless it moves or we move our head away quickly from an eye approaching object before we recognize what it actually is.

Visual memory in some birds is very important at an early age in order to recognize the parents. Thus, extensive visual and associative brain areas must be present at birth. Newly hatched ducks and geese attach themselves to and follow the very first object they see move and store this memory in their brains. This is usually the mother who now will not lose their offsprings and can guide and train them through their first days and weeks of life. In the laboratory it has been shown that this object can basically be anything including a person. These little ducks will then follow the person "thinking" this is their mother. Some birds can hide hundreds of seeds in different locations and still find them again after some time. Homing pigeons use visual orientation and memories (in addition to the sun and magnetic fields) to find their way home since it has been found that they fly often along landmarks like thruways. Pigeons have even been shown that they can be trained to memorize and distinguish between the paintings of Monet and Picasso. Birds can even exhibit some abstract thinking. Rooks which are members of the crow family have been observed to get water from a jar with a water level too low to drink from by placing nearby pebbles into this jar to raise the water level. Interestingly, they will start with the largest pebbles because these would raise the level fastest. Certain crow Jays have been observed to watch other birds in order to protect their hidden foods. These birds will store food in a hiding place and will look around if other birds are present. If yes, they will come back after a while when no birds are around, recover the food and store it in a different place to avoid other birds from "stealing" their food. On a "smartness" scale birds seem to be just a bit below the apes and way above most other animals.

Some dinosaurs which seem to be the ancestors of birds (not reptiles) had in addition to their brains in the head a large cluster of nerve cells (second brain??) at the beginning of the tail which helped these animals to control lower body and tail movement more efficiently.

Vision and its interpretation of an object or another animal by the brain play a major role in the interaction among animals of the same species or among species. Size elicits prey catching or predator avoidance movements in most animals. Toads have been shown to try to catch small objects while avoiding larger ones. When male animals like wolves or deer within a group establish their rank order, size plays an important role. Animals look closely at each other and estimate the size of the opponent with the smaller animal most often retreating and avoiding the fight. Color also plays a role. Among birds, female birds taking care of the eggs will have bland colors as not to be recognized quickly while the male has brighter colors to be recognized faster and to detract predators when flying from the nest. Birds will sometimes display a distraction maneuver: they will fly away from the nest in such a way as to give the predator the visual impression that they are hurt by not using one wing properly. They lure the predator away from the nest and then fly off quickly. Colors will also play a role in mating. The darker breasted a male swallow the more it is attractive to females. When scientists observed breeding behavior of dark and light breasted swallows and then covered the dark colors on the dark breasted and painted dark paint on the light breasted birds, females changed their mating behavior neglecting the now "lighter" and preferring the "darker" males.

Vision also allows us to obtain some insight into the "workings" of an animal's brain. Visual experiments have shown that animals can actually do some "abstract" thinking and some rudimentary mathematics. When chimps were shown one apple placed into one box and five apples into another box, they would invariably go for the box with five apples. Similarly, robins were shown where various numbers of worms were stored in a hole and then allowed to feed – they would invariably fly to the hole with the most worms. The researchers feel that they can identify numbers up to twelve. When chicks were hatched and imprinted with one or five objects they would always follow either the one object or five objects. If the five object imprinted birds were confronted with either two or four objects they would follow the four objects which are closer to the five objects they were imprinted with.

The human feature of visual self-recognition (see before) – recognizing one's own face in the mirror- can be measured by placing, for instance, a colored spot unbeknownst to the person on the face and the subject is then shown a mirror. The subject – starting in humans at an age of about two years – will touch the mark on his or her face indicating that he or she is recognizing his or her own face in the mirror. This test can also be done in animals and most animals fail the test except higher apes like chimpanzees and orangutans (with most gorillas failing the test) and interestingly also elephants and dolphins.

At the end, it might be interesting to note that animals also possess senses which humans have but which are either poorly developed or are even absent. Below are a few examples of such special senses.

It was already mentioned that animals rely heavily on smell. However, microbiologists recently discovered that even bacteria communicate by "smell" (or "taste"). Pathogenic or disease causing bacteria do not seem to attack the tissues in the body until they have multiplied and have reached a critical number. So – how do these bacteria know when that number has been reached? They seem to do this by sending out chemicals which tell the individual bacteria that this number is reached and they can now start attacking the host. Ants are masters in the "language" of smell. A few molecules of a chemical secreted by these blind creatures along their way will guide them back later on to the nest as well as serve as a communication with other ants to tell them that they found no or lots of food. We all have this experienced in that one ant in the kitchen which found a bread crump will result within minutes in ten or twenty ants arriving. Moths can smell a few molecules of a chemical or pheromone which has been secreted by another moth a mile away to find a mate. Mosquitoes can detect the exhaled carbon dioxide of a human to find their next blood meal. All of this is accomplished with no brain as in the case of the bacteria or a brain which is the size of the dot at the end of this sentence. Snakes can sniff with their forked tongues which collect particles wafting in the air. The tongue is then dipped into special pits in the roof of the mouth where the odors are processed and signals are sent to the brain. Salmons find their way back from the ocean to the place of their birth in a small river to breed by using smell (and other senses - see below). Each of these places has an unique smell which has been imprinted to the newly hatched fish at birth and during the first days of life to be remembered for all those years when these fish are living in the ocean far away from their birthplace. The blood hound can trace the footsteps of a human even after days have passed and in some cases even after it had rained. The nasal chambers of these dogs which are larger than those of other dogs collect scents more efficiently so that even minute amounts can be detected and identified. The folds of wrinkled flesh under the lips and neck help further to catch stray scent chemicals from nearby branches. Dogs are used today for security reasons to sniff out hidden explosives, to find people buried in a collapsed building and perhaps medically in the future as well since it has been shown that dogs can detect if individuals will soon experience an epileptic episode or can smell if the urine comes from a healthy individual or a cancer patient.

But animals have senses more delicately developed than those in humans or such senses which are even absent in humans.

The lowly beetle has specialized receptors at the eye which detect polarized light from the sky (which humans cannot see) and which serves as a guide to help it move around. The electric eel is a fish which can generate powerful electric shocks, which it uses for hunting and self-defense. It possesses three special organs that produce electricity. Some of these organs are used for electrolocation or orientation. Other organs send out electrical signals to communicate with other eels, to find a mate and to locate prey. Other organs produce high-voltage electricity which will stun or kill the prey. Such shocks can be quite dangerous to humans.

The electromagnetic fields of the earth which humans cannot detect are being used by animals for orientation and to find prey. Sharks possess special receptors numbering in the hundreds to thousands to detect these fields for their orientation and navigation. Since all living organisms including smaller fish produce such fields as well, they can be detected by sharks even from a fish which hides in the sand. Since boats also generate sometimes such a field, sharks are known to attack the boat in the mistaken belief it is prey. Certain species of birds which migrate often over many hundred of miles employ these fields during their flights for finding their way. In addition to the mentioned visual clues, they use the electromagnetic field of the earth. This field varies in strength depending on the latitudes and birds seem to be able to detect and use these differences for their orientation. It has been shown that these birds have a neural connection between the eye and a special part of the brain thought to be responsible for such perception which might suggest that they actually "see" the electromagnetic field of the earth. Similarly, turtles and salmons use their eyes to feed but also the magnetic field around the earth to find their way "home" to their breeding grounds. Salmons find the mouth of the river in which they were born (and then smell takes them up-stream to their birthplace to spawn as well as to their graves since after mating and laying the eggs both male and female fish die and their decaying and disintegrating bodies provide food for their offsprings). The homing sense of pigeons has been well known for years and has been exploited during wars and other occasions. It is still uncertain how pigeons do this navigational feat but it has been proposed that they use the sun and the magnetic field of the earth.

Boas and vipers possess temperature-sensitive organs between the eyes and nostrils which allow them to sense the body heat of their prey. Since there is one of these organs located on each side of the head, snakes have depth perception and can strike with accuracy even if it is dark.

Mice and rats have whiskers around their snouts. They use these long hairs (vibrissae) in a way like blind people use their canes. By whisking the hairs across objects these animals can then form an image of their shapes.

Animals use "sonar" or echolocation. A sonar system basically consists of pulses of sound waves which are sent into space and when hitting an object are reflected back to their source. These reflected waves allow the sender to determine the existence of and distance to an object.

Some animals send out waves from special organs of their heads and then receive the reflected waves with their ears. Since the two ears are slightly apart, reflected waves arrive at slightly different times at each ear. This difference allows them to detect the exact location of an object. Bats flying in a pitch dark night send out such sound waves with a frequency of about 75 000 vibrations per second (humans can ultimately detect about 20 000) and can easily locate a meal of a flying insect. Whales diving into the dark depth of the ocean use sonar as well. They send out "clicks" or special sound waves and their reflections tell the whales where to swim but also where to find food. It has been suggested that the sonar system of the whales is superior to the most sophisticated sonar systems of the human engineers. It has also been suggested that the human sonar system as used by marine vessels might interfere with that of the whales and causes harm like mass beaching of whales and other marine animals.

Animals seem to sense that other animals of the same species are sick. Whether this is done by smell or vision or other senses is unclear. But it has been observed that they often shun and avoid sick animals or even attack or kill them. Wild lobsters of one species usually live together in small groups in a den while sick lobsters have been found to be shunned and are forced to live a solitary existence. In laboratory experiments, healthy lobsters were brought together with virus infected lobsters and were found to avoid the sick lobsters. In the laboratory, it can be often observed that laboratory rats housed together in a cage will live together peacefully but start attacking and eating a sick or dying mate.

What about plants? Do plants have photosensitive cells or even "eyes" and can they "see"? No, they cannot see – but they not only need "light" to grow and reproduce but can also "detect" light. First, they need the energy of the electromagnetic waves or "light" for photosynthesis where the plants convert carbon dioxide into cellulose and other chemicals necessary for them to grow and multiply. The plants then expel oxygen which animals and humans need to breathe and live. It has been proposed that plants actually made animal and human life possible. The original atmosphere of the earth billions of years ago contained no oxygen but – among other gases – carbon dioxide. Growing algae in the oceans would now use the carbon dioxide and produce oxygen which would slowly accumulate in the water making it possible for the development of fish. Later on, the oxygen would escape the water and fill the air with more and more oxygen. This made it possible for oxygen breathing organisms to develop on land which would finally culminate in the evolution of the human race. Thus, we own our existence to those lowly algae and other land plants to provide us with our oxygen. Second, plants do respond to light. It is a well known observation that plants usually grow towards light. This process is called phototropism. Here, plants have special light receptors which respond to light and, interestingly, some plants will respond preferentially to blue or red light. Light causes the formation of certain growth hormones (called auxins) on the dark side of a plant which causes these cells to become more elongated bending the plant towards the light (roots, in contrast, seem to follow gravity). However, some plants do it the other way around – they exhibit negative phototropism or growing towards the dark region. Leaves respond to the presence and the movement of the sun (a process called heliotropism). They often let their leaves droop during the night and raise them with sunrise. Sunflowers actually move their leaves and flowers during the day and follow the course of the sun. Plants also respond to seasons or show photoperiodism. Here, the plants sense the lengths of the days or the daily photoperiod. They contain special chemicals (like phytochromes or cryptochromes) which tell them when to flower or not. Some will flower on short while others only on long days. Plants that will only flower when the night is long will not do so if a bright light is briefly shone onto them during darkness. However, moonlight or lightning is not of sufficient brightness or duration to interrupt their flowering. Third, many flowering plants, e.g. orchids in particular, have used the vision of other creatures to help them to reproduce. They have developed all kinds of brilliant colors and color combinations to attract insects which then feed on their nectar and pollinate the germ cells for procreation. Thus, plants depend on light and use it for growth, multiplication and survival – and indirectly support fish, birds, animals and humans by producing the oxygen without which life is impossible.

Studies of the eyes and brains and the visual processes of the animal kingdom have also given us some clues and hints how our eyes, brains and the vision process slowly evolved over millions and millions of years until it reached our present state. It most likely started out with some very simple and primitive structures which could only detect and respond to light. These photosensitive structures became then more and more refined and finally connected to more and more nerve cells to bring vision into existence as we know it today. Improved vision apparently helped these organisms to better survive and to reproduce. Thus, let us trace the development of our eyes and then that of our visual brain areas through the animal kingdom in order to get some idea how they slowly evolved.

The amoeba is a one celled organism (no photosensitive or nerve cells) but still responds to light. It moves away from intense light but gets attracted to weak light. This is done by increasing the thickness of the pseudopods (the little extensions of the cell wall which moves the microbe). Apparently, light sensitive chemicals must exist in this tiny cell which respond to light and transmit this information to the cell wall. This movement is called phototaxis and is probably the very first origin of our eyes. Such light sensitive chemicals were identified in the hydra which has no eyes but will contract rapidly into a ball when exposed to sudden bright light. Researchers have found that hydras respond to light using two proteins (which are interestingly closely related to those also found in our own eyes). The first light detecting cell most likely originated with another one celled creature like a euglena which contained one photosensitive cell which was connected to a tail or flagellum allowing it to move towards light. The next step was perhaps the multi-cellular marine ragworm Platynereis. This tiny creature possesses two cells that respond to light and are sometimes called "proto-eyes". One is a pigment cell and one a light-sensitive cell. The pigment cell absorbs light and casts a shadow over the light-sensitive or photoreceptor cell. The shape of the shadow varies according to the position of the light source. The photoreceptor cell then converts this light signal into electricity, sending it as a signal along a nerve that connects to a band of cells endowed with thin hairs that beat to displace water and that then propel the worm.

Other worms increased the number of these photosensitive cells and the common earth worm possesses such a number of such cells - called ocelli - all over its bodies which make the worm notice and respond quickly to light. Such a worm when unearthed will avoid light and move hurriedly back into the earth

Such photosensitive cells started to cluster at first on the outside of a body. They then slowly started to move inside the organism to be better protected and to form the first primitive "pit eye". As the pit deepened the number of photoreceptive cells increased inside the pit. The pit allowed for a more directional light reception since only frontal light would enter the pit allowing the organism to sense the origin of the light source. Such early "eyes" are seen in the mollusk nautilus.

The opening of this pit was then closed with a membrane which started to divide into two layers like in some snails. More advanced land snails have two primitive eyes each located at the tip of its tentacles (albeit eye structures vary greatly among these snails). This allows the snail to move the eyes around for better vision. The schematic diagram of an advanced snail eye showing the dermal cornea (A), the eye cornea (B), the lens (C), the retina (D) and the optic nerve (E) are shown below:

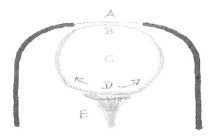

Figure 40

Interestingly, the snail can retract its eye for protection into the tentacle.

The outer membrane (A in above diagram) became later a true cornea while the inner layer (B in the above diagram) most likely became an iris.

All what was left was the development of the ciliary body surrounding the lens. This occurred slowly and the frog eye already sports such a muscle. From now on all the basic structures of the eye had been developed and can be found quite low at the bottom of the evolutionary tree. From now on the location and structure of the eye only became more varied and specialized as higher animals evolved in different environments. These special adaptations allowed each organism to survive and reproduce in its particular surroundings.

Recently, it was suggested that the aquatic hydra had evolved about 600 million years ago. This would indicate that the first light responding proteins also originated at this time. Similarly, some of the genes like the gene Pax6 which are responsible in forming advanced eyes have been detected in very early organisms. Based on the genetic composition necessary to build more advanced eyes, researchers have estimated that it should only take evolution 364,000 years to move from photosensitive cells to a primitive eye. It would take somewhat longer if one adds to the development of the eye that of the brain – but nature had millions and millions of years and a vast number of different genetic combinations available to do so. This progress was accelerated as more and more organisms originated and became more diversified and complex. This fostered the development of more advanced eyes needed to catch prey or to avoid predators.

Less is known about the development of the brain and its visual central areas except that it must also have started from one single nerve cell. But how did this cell come into existence which upon stimulation by a chemical (a neurotransmitter) would conduct an electrical impulse from one end to the other end of the cell and would there release a chemical which would initiate another nerve impulse or activate a muscle? The origin of our neurons and brains might have started – as some scientists believe - with the sponges which do not have nerve cells but posses in their DNA many of the genes necessary to form nerve cells. The existence of this was proven when these special genes were incorporated into the DNA of frogs and were expressed by forming actual nerve cells. The question can be asked: if they have these genes why do they not form nerve cells? Apparently, other genes are also necessary to form nerve cells which had not yet developed. Nevertheless, sponges do respond to touch which causes some movement. The next step was most likely partial expression of these genes in the jelly fish. Some researchers speculate that this occurred in the cells of their bellies which can both detect physical contact (like a nerve cell) and can contract (like a muscle cell) in response. Genes in such cells might then have developed into specialized genes which would now manufacture either nerve or muscle cells. This might have occurred in the ragworm Platynereis, a still living "fossil". This marine worm has primitive nerve cells which respond to the activity of photoreceptors cells (see above) and which control a band of cilias which move and propel the worm. From these primitive "nerve cells" of the ragworm, organisms started to develop more of these nerve cells and accumulated them in clusters and networks. This can be seen in the hydra which has a number of nerve cells which form a network spreading over its entire body with a higher density in the head and the foot. These cells also show some specialization in that some respond to touch and others to chemicals. Interestingly, hydras continuously form these nerve cells from precursor cells during their life time and the precursor cells can migrate to any part of the body to form new nerve cells (feats which the human body cannot or only do very poorly). Flatworms have a more distinct nerve net connected by two long cords and a slight accumulation in the head (white lines). The pictures below show a hydra (left) and a flatworm (right):

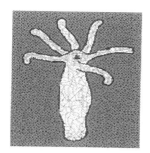 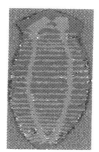

Figure 41

Slowly more nerve cells developed and accumulated and aplasia, the sea slug, has already about 20 000 nerve cells in its frontal area or its brain. In the ocean, the number of nerve cells started to increase rapidly among species and the octopus sports about 300 000 000 such cells (although its brain is oddly wrapped around the esophagus – a side line of evolution which other animals did not follow). Researchers believe that this creature is one of the most intelligent marine animals. On land, the development seemed to have developed more slowly and sometimes differently. Worms on land, like the worm C. elegans has a condensed ring of about 302 neurons near the head which could be called a "pre-brain". They respond to light and control movements of the worm as well. Over time, more cells started to cluster together at the front of the organisms and formed more and more complex brains. Among the insects, the bee brain has been estimated to contain about 850 000 neurons. As brains became more complex, they began to sub-divide their jobs and to form special brain areas each with its own function but nevertheless always in contact with each other and working together. Each area would now be in charge of breathing, heart beats, movements, digestive processes and sensations including vision as well as certain acquired, albeit primitive memories.

For visual purposes, the connections of the photosensitive cells and their nerve cells in the eye with more complex neuronal networks in the brains allowed these organisms to perceive not only light or darkness but also visual pictures, detect colors and store visual memories. Roughly, this development can be divided into three major parts (although overlaps did occur during this development). The reptile brain is one of the "oldest" and perhaps the most fundamental brain. It controls all the basic functions of the body like the heart and respiration as well as vision and movements. The visual area in these animals is mostly specialized in "seeing" but not very much in "interpreting" an object as outlined above. Later on, lower mammals started to add another part to this already existing structure which is commonly called the limbic brain. Here, emotions, judgments and decisions are processed and memories can be stored, interpreted and recalled. The next step was the addition of a neocortex which was very primitive and small at first but began to grow in size and structure with the primates and humans showing the largest and most detailed structure. In particular the frontal lobe started to increase in size. This allowed for a better comprehension of the environment and a more detailed and appropriate response pattern. Visual objects were more clearly seen and could be better analyzed, interpreted, stored and later on used and recalled. In humans, the cortex is mostly responsible for sensations and abstract thinking with the frontal lobe being what has often been called the "controller" of our behavior.

Thus, living conditions and survival in certain environments drove the development of the eyes and brains always suiting the life style of a particular organism and insuring its best survival chances and reproduction possibilities. It is uncertain if better and more developed eyes did lead to more complex visual brain structures and areas or if the development of more complex brain structures fostered the evolution of more refined eyes.

The study of the visual system of animals is not only of general biological interest but has provided us with valuable clues as to the origin and development of the human visual system and studies with laboratory animals e.g. rats, cats and monkeys have given us and are still providing us with major insights into the basis and functioning of the human visual system which is so essential to our daily lives. Studies with animals have already allowed us and will still allow us in the future to find newer and better treatments and cures for ocular disorders and diseases. Thus, we have to be grateful and thankful to all the animals.

A Look Into the Future

Introduction. Over the last decades significant progress in treating eye problems and preventing or delaying vision loss due to diseases of the eye has been made. For instance, in 2002 about 2000 cases of cancer of the eye were recorded. Five decades ago, this would have resulted most likely in 2000 deaths. However, newer drug and other treatment modalities reduced this figure to 200 or the vast majority of patients did not have to die. Similar results can be cited with other ocular problems including age related macular degeneration which five decades ago would have resulted in severe vision loss or blindness in all patients. Newer drug therapies can now markedly slow down visual impairment and preserve vision for a much longer time. But still more has to be done. Scientists and physicians are trying to improve existing treatments and to develop novel and even more effective therapies. This is being done on many fronts including patients, animals, isolated ocular tissues and individual cells. This research is a combined effort of many disciplines involving chemistry, physics, genetics, biochemistry, physiology, microbiology, pharmacology and ophthalmology. It might, thus, be interesting to look at some of these experimental and theoretical approaches which are currently under investigation to prevent and restore vision loss. Some of these might bear fruit within the very near future while others might take a bit longer.

Physics. People with very low vision who are not helped with ordinary eye glasses can be furnished with small telescopes. These can be mounted on regular eye glasses but many individuals feel that this is very inconvenient and unsightly. However, they can also be implanted into the cornea directly where they are much less noticeable.

The problem can be that the body tries to reject the foreign material. To circumvent this problem, researches used a tooth from a patient, ground it down, drilled a hole into the remainder, inserted the lenses and implanted it into the eye which was much better tolerated. This gives rise to hope for individuals who had trouble with the older devices.

For people who are blind technology is being used to restore some vision – often using unexpected avenues. One approach consists of attaching a tiny camera to the frame of eye glasses which would send electric signals to an electrode chip sewn to the back wall of the eye. This chip then creates electrical impulses which it would pass on to retinal nerve cells and which in turn would send these signals to the visual area of the brain. This approach has already been tried in five blind people who reported to see spots and lines of light. In a similar procedure, a computer processed the presented data and sent electrical impulses to electrodes which had been surgically implanted directly on the visual cortex areas of the brain. First test results showed that subjects had recovered some vision. A patient who had been completely blind reported to actually see landmarks of shape and shadow.

Another approach uses the plasticity of the brain where one area of the brain can assume the task which ordinarily would be performed by another area. In this case, the "feeling" area is trained to "see". A multitude of pins attached to the skin of the back of a subject were activated to present a figure. The subject reported that he/she could actually visualize the pin pricks as this particular figure. This procedure is now being refined by several research teams. Similarly, a dense array of pins has been developed which can be made to vibrate individually on the finger of a blind person. Printed material is scanned by an array of photocells which are coupled individually to these pins. Again, the individual felt the image of the letters on his/her fingers and could assemble a visual image of the word. Reading tests with this procedure by blind subjects have been reported to recognize about 30 correct words per minute. More recently, the tongue which has many delicate receptors on its surface has been employed. A camera projected a picture to a chip or a plastic film with sensors and electrodes which were placed on the tongue. When activated the chip sent individual electrical impulses to the tongue which stimulated these receptors and sent electrical impulses via nerves to the brain. Early experiments have shown that individuals could "see", albeit in a rudimentary way, the projected pictures. Individual patients actually responded so well that such a patient was actually able to catch a ball. This patient reported: *the physician rolled a tennis ball towards me and a small point on my tongue started to tickle. The closer the ball came to me, the bigger the point became – and then all of a sudden I had a picture of a ball in my head and I could actually catch the ball.* In all of these experiments it is attempted to train areas in the brain which normally respond to other receptors to start to change and to "see". That this approach is feasible has been shown experimentally in animals. For instance, when the optic nerve of young ferrets was surgically removed from the visual area and directed to the auditory area, these animals after some training could see albeit not normal and showed "visual" activity in this brain area. While these experiments and possibilities not only show promise for blind patients, they also hold promise for stroke patients or individuals with accidental brain injuries where certain visual areas have been damaged, stopped to function properly and caused visual problems.

Researchers also work on a car for the blind which follows the voice commands of the driver. The driver is being guided by vibrating bells about the experimental environment which is constantly being screened by lasers.

Thus, progress in physics and electro technology opens up a number of new avenues to help the blind or severely vision impaired.

Drug therapy. Advances are being made to develop more effective ways to use existing drugs or to invent even more effective drugs with less adverse reactions. In the first place, the ophthalmologist already has available – mostly during the last five decades – a number of quite effective medications to treat various ocular problems. Unfortunately, drops applied to the eye have two drawbacks – drugs do not penetrate deep enough into the eye such as the retina and they are short lived which requires often frequent applications (which many patients forget to do and thus diminish the effectiveness of their medications). In addition, drugs applied to the outer eye will quickly move through the nasal passage into the nose and mouth and will be absorbed into the body causing adverse reactions in the body. The ophthalmologist must sometimes inject the drug around or into the eye in order to treat the innermost part of the eye which is emotional upsetting to the patient and can cause infections. New methodologies are now applied to remedy some of these problems. For instance, drugs are encapsulated in tiny capsules of a special polymer (these nano packets range from about 10-1000 nanometer – a nanometer is a billionth of a meter) which penetrate the eye well and slowly release the drug over longer periods of time. First trials are very promising and will reduce the number of applications and sometimes eliminate injections. Only 15% of a common antiglaucoma drug applied to the rabbit eye was found inside the eye and it disappeared after about 5 hours. In contrast, 75 % of the same drug applied in nano particles was found inside the eye and was still detectable after 2 days. Human trials are in progress. Among new drug developments, monoclonal antibodies and antisense drugs seem to be the most promising. Monoclonal antibodies are antibodies which are not produced by the body but in the laboratory from single human cells. They are very specific for their interaction with microbes but also for certain chemicals in the body or the eye. Some are already been used with great success in the treatment of the "wet" form of macular degeneration or AMD like ranibizumab (-mab means **m**onoclonal **antib**ody). This drug selectively interferes with the vascular endothelial growth factor or VEGF which is necessary for the formation of new blood vessels. This interference reduces the amount of VEGF and decreases the formation of the unwanted new blood vessels in the "wet" form. More drugs of this type are on the horizon which will be more selective and thus produce no or only minimal adverse reactions. Antisense drugs are very effective when a specific gene known to cause a particular disease forms a harmful peptide or protein (the normal sequence is: a gene of DNA or **D**eoxyribose **N**ucleic **A**cid forms a specific RNA or **R**ibose **N**ucleic **A**cid molecule which in turn forms a specific peptide or protein). The antisense drug is a very short version of a nucleic acid sequence which binds to the site of RNA which produces this peptide or protein. The binding of the antisense drug then prevents formation of this compounds. Some of these antisense drugs are already used in the treatment of the "wet" form of AMD like pegaptanib which in this case prevents the synthesis of VEGF and subsequently the formation of unwanted blood vessels. Similar drugs are being developed against viruses and ocular cancers with a very bright future for such patients.

Sometimes nature comes to our help. It has been found that deep sea fish living in utter darkness use chlorophyll (which actually only has been found in plants with these fish being the first reported exception) in their eyes to help them to see in this darkness. Recent experiments have used eye drops containing chlorophyll to affect vision in rats and rabbits and indeed vision could be markedly improved in these animals.

Nerve cells in the eye and brain do not usually regenerate or repair themselves after injury. However, when the lens of an animal with a damaged optic nerve was scratched, it was observed – not surprisingly – that white blood cells would aggregate around the lens to help repair the damage. But, more surprisingly, it was also observed that the optic nerve of these eyes started to regenerate and grow. Researchers could isolate a special protein (called (oncomodulin) which in other experiments showed that its application to an eye with an injured optic nerve indeed made this nerve grow. This is not only important for the eye but could have tremendous applications for other bodily nerves as well. This might help individuals with low vision but could also benefit e.g. stroke victims to re-grow lost neurons. These are just a few examples and the next decade should bring some major breakthroughs.

Stem cells. Stem cells offer a possibility to perhaps restore already destroyed tissue and its function. Stem cells are special cells in the human body which have no tissue characteristics but can develop into any tissue cell. Thus, a stem cell injected into a heart will become a heart cell while the same cell if it would have been injected into the liver, would have become a liver cell. Stem cells can become a cell of any tissue and start to grow and multiply. These cells can be obtained from embryonic tissue but can also be harvested from a person (adult stem cells) since everyone carries some stem cells in his or her body. They can be isolated from their sources and injected into a recipient or can be grown in a Petri dish under proper conditions to form a layer or the beginning of any tissue.

A number of research teams already reported success in restoring damaged and nonfunctioning ocular tissue with these cells. For instance, such cells were transplanted into the eyes of mice and found to be accepted and to migrate into the right places of the eye and to form healthy retinal cells. In another experiment, mice which suffered from a genetic disorder and which would show retinal degeneration were treated with an injection of stem cells. It was found that this significantly preserved their vision. All this is very encouraging and offers hope for humans with retinal problems. The first human experiments and trials are already under way. For instance, a research team from England reported in 2008 that they had used stem cells in almost completely blind people which were now able to read large print after treatment. These were patients who had suffered from chemical burns which had rendered their corneas opaque with blood vessels growing across it. The researchers used a plastic material on which they grew these stem cells into a cornea and then implanted it into the eye. The research team said *"before the surgery the patients were barely able to recognize when someone was waving a hand in front of their face but we have restored their vision to the point they can read three to four lines down the eye chart."* In 2009, another research team reported that they treated three patients who were blind in one eye. They obtained stem cells from the healthy eyes and cultured them on extended wear contact lenses for ten days. The surfaces of the patients' corneas were then cleaned and the contact lenses inserted. Within 10 to 14 days the stem cells began to recolonize and repair the damaged cornea. Vision was partially restored. While repair of the outer parts of the eye is progressing nicely, it is still difficult to repair damaged inner parts of the eye in particular the retina. However, recent studies in animals with macular damage have shown that it might be possible to repair and regenerate a damaged retina in animals. Thus, stem cell research might indeed open up new and very promising avenues to restore ocular damage and to provide such individuals with vision again.

Genetics. Another promising field is genetics. Interestingly, genetics is a very young science. Although general genetics was known for a long time as it was used mostly by breeders to selectively breed animals and plants. A major breakthrough in understanding how genetics actually works came with the work of Gregor Mendel (about 1850) who discovered the basic principles of heredity which are known today as Mendel's laws. The next breakthrough occurred with the discovery of DNA by Crick and Watson (about1955) as the genetic material of our cells and body. From there on our knowledge of genetics literally exploded and recently the entire human genome was deciphered. Scientists today have a good idea how genes work and how to use them beneficially in medicine. Thus, when we talk about genes and genetic diseases and genetic engineering, all this has only occurred roughly within the last two to three decades. The long molecules of DNA in our cell nucleus are composed of many special segments called genes which code for or determine the formation of specific proteins which are used to make cells and to function as catalysts to synthesize our biochemicals in the body. If a gene is missing or malfunctioning, then a special protein will not be made or made in an abnormal form. The result is a disturbance of the normal state of a cell. If this disturbance is significant, diseases arise. This might be seen right at birth or might be expressed later on in Life. Such a malfunction of one or more genes can be inherited but can also be caused during the aging process or due to environmental influences such as radiation, certain chemicals and also some drugs (in particular if used during pregnancy). Today, we know many of the genes which make up our healthy eye. We also find out gradually which missing or malfunctioning genes cause certain ocular diseases.

Thus, theoretically it can now be proposed to insert the healthy gene into the DNA of an individual who lacks this gene. This would mean that the disease is now cured. This sounds very logical and simple but it presents a tremendous experimental challenge. The human DNA contains thousands of genes and each gene contains hundreds of individual chemicals. Below is schematically shown a very small part of a DNA molecule (which actually is twisted into a double helix) with the letters each indicating a specific gene (one from the father and one from the mother depicted in italics:

```
----========----========----========----==============----=====-------
   A       B        C        D'       E        F        G
```

```
----========----========----========----==============----=====-------
   A       B        C        D        E        F        G
```

The defective or missing gene has first to be found among the thousands of genes (let it be D'). Then a healthy gene (D) has to be isolated and inserted into the right place of the DNA (for instance D between C and E and not between E and G) of such a patient. This presents enormous challenges. Scientists, however, have developed methods which appear promising. It has been found that certain genes can be experimentally eliminated from the DNA of animals (e.g. mice or rats). These animals (called knock-out animals) will then display certain pathological problems some of which resemble human diseases. The eliminated gene can be inserted into harmless viruses which are known to introduce their genetic material into that of the host cell. After the virus has been given to the animal, it can be observed if the gene has been properly inserted and if the problems have been corrected. Scientists have made tremendous progress using these (and other) procedures in animals. For instance, healthy mice have only receptor proteins in the retina which are sensitive to blue and green hues. They cannot see red hues. These mice were treated with the human gene which makes the red light responding protein. After treatment, the engineered mice could now easily discriminate a bright red light. All these experiments bode well for human patients and a number of human trials have already been performed and more are under way. But there are still many ethical and medical problems, for instance, will the virus per se or a gene inserted in the wrong place cause unforeseen problems and lead to more harm or even death of such subjects..

In case of ocular diseases, progress has been made. A number of genetic abnormalities have been detected and identified in individuals with various ocular problems. Patients with Leber's Congenital Amaurosis will become blind at an early age because they have a faulty gene which makes photoreceptor cells that do not work properly. This gene was recently identified as RPE65. Fortunately, some dogs are known to suffer from a genetic disorder which will also leads to early blindness. Recent research in these animals has identified the culprit as a faulty gene called RPE65 or the same gene which was not functioning properly in the human patients. When this faulty gene was replaced with the healthy gene, the vision of these dogs was slowly restored. Similar experiments were done in chickens which also can have this faulty gene and are born blind. Injection of the healthy gene into the egg of such chickens caused the hatching of chickens with almost normal vision. The first human trials are now under way. Genetic engineering has also been successful in animals to restore or originate color vision. Two adult, male squirrel monkeys, named Dalton and Sam, were found to be red-green color-blind since birth (a condition that similarly affects humans but more males than females). Five months after researchers injected human genes responsible for this color vision into the monkeys' eyes, the duo could see red as if they had always had this ability. While some scientists are convinced that this is an effective and safe procedure, other scientists are concerned about unforeseen harmful possibilities. However, it is hoped that the benefits to the patients will be greater than any unforeseen adverse reactions. The final decision maker will almost be the patient who after careful explanations of the benefits and risks has to say yes or no.

Magic. Everybody knows fairy tales about invisible characters, individuals who can become invisible and the movies about the "invisible man". This is magic and unreal – but perhaps not. Vision means that light waves have to be reflected off the surface of objects and to reach our eyes where these objects are then finally seen in our brains. Depending on the wavelength, objects can appear white or colored. If the light waves are completely absorbed, the object appears black. If light waves are not reflected and are not absorbed, then we do not see anything. Looking across empty space, means we see nothing. What would happen if the light waves would not be reflected or absorbed by an object – well, the object would be there but we would not see it. Impossible – no, scientists have developed "metamaterials" which can do just this. Objects made out of these "metamaterials" do not absorb or reflect light waves and the object is invisible. Scientists indeed are working on this project and have made first progress in actually "hiding" an object or a person (unfortunately, the person inside such an invisible "cloak" could not see out of it either). Of course, the military are quite interested in such materials for obvious reasons. But in more scientific and medical terms, such "metamaterials" can also concentrate light and serve as a "superlens" providing scientist with the possibility to develop a "supermicroscope" – surpassing our sophisticated electron microscope by many measures and allowing us to study ever more delicate details of nature and the human body including the eye.

Conclusion. A number of new developments show great promise – however, as with all new developments it is imprudent to expect the final result to become available tomorrow. Some of them might turn out to be impractical, some might take a long time to become available than originally thought and some – by surprise – might make it into medicine much earlier than expected. Nevertheless, progress has been made and beneficial results have been obtained to be optimistic in keeping our eyes and brains more healthy and helping patients who are severely vision impaired or blind.

Biography

Wolfgang H. Vogel, Ph.D. completed his training at the University in Stuttgart, Germany, and the National Institutes of Health, Bethesda and carried out extensive research and taught full time Pharmacology in particular Ocular Pharmacology and Physiology at Jefferson Medical College of Thomas Jefferson and part time at the Osteopathic College of Medicine of New Jersey, the College of Podiatric Medicine and the Pennsylvania College of Optometry in Philadelphia. He was full Professor and acting Chairman of the Department of Pharmacology at Thomas Jefferson University. He served on a large number of national and international scientific committees and lectured on his research widely abroad. He published over 300 scientific abstracts and papers, 12 major chapters in 4 Clinical Handbooks and 7 books on drug development, general and ocular pharmacology and the history of vision and ocular medicine. He is now retired and lives in Florida but is still busy writing and lecturing.

Dr. Steven Pascucci M.D. graduated from Jefferson Medical College in Philadelphia, PA. He performed an internship in Internal Medicine at The Lankenau Hospital, Philadelphia and a residency in Ophthalmology at The University of South Florida, Tampa. He was a partner and member of the board of directors of Northeastern Eye Institute, Scranton, PA. He has served on the Bausch & Lomb Medical Advisory Board and was the first surgeon in the Unites States to use the Schwind-Corriazo Pendular Microkeratome. Currently, he is the Medical Director of Eye Consultants of Bonita Springs, Bonita Springs, FL. His practice focuses upon corneal, refractive and anterior segment surgery as well as anterior segment complications. He is a member of the editorial board of Review of Ophthalmology, Refractive Eyecare for Ophthalmologists and editor of Review of Ophthalmology Online. He also holds the academic position of Affiliate Assistant Professor of Ophthalmology in the Department of Ophthalmology of The University of South Florida in Tampa, FL.